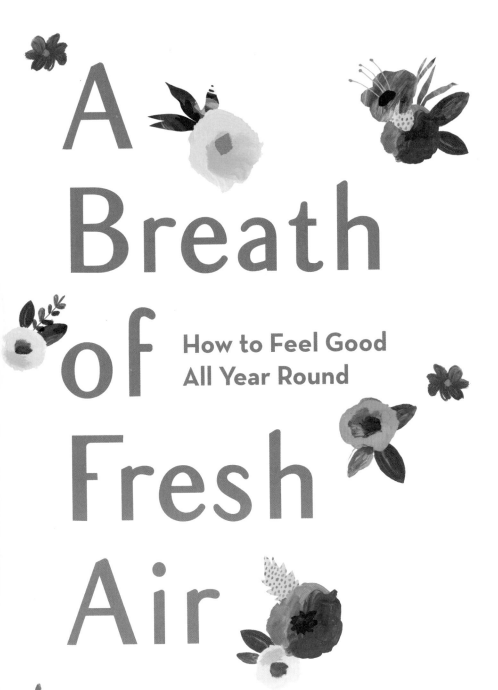

A Breath of Fresh Air

How to Feel Good All Year Round

For my dad, Ian, who found wonder in life's simple pleasures.

First published in the United Kingdom in 2020 by
National Trust Books
43 Great Ormond Street
London
WC1N 3HZ

An imprint of Pavilion Books Group Ltd

Volume © National Trust Books, 2020
Text by Rebecca Frank, © National Trust Books, 2020

ISBN: 9781911358893

A CIP catalogue record for this book is available from the British Library.

10 9 8 7 6 5 4 3 2 1

Reproduction by Rival Colour Ltd, UK
Printed and bound by 1010 Printing International Ltd, China

This book can be ordered direct from the publisher at the website:
www.pavilionbooks.com, or try your local bookshop. Also available at
National Trust shops or www.nationaltrustbooks.co.uk

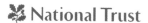 National Trust

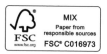

A Breath of Fresh Air

How to Feel Good All Year Round

Rebecca Frank

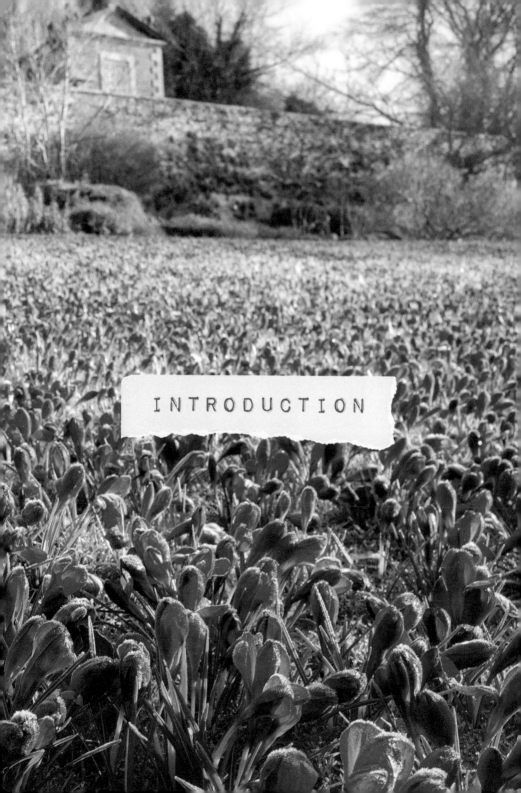

INTRODUCTION

It's easy to go through life on autopilot. To follow routines and to-do lists, just getting on with what we do without really thinking too much about it. Yet if we slow down a little and consider more carefully how we spend our time, why we're doing something and how to get more from our experiences, it could help us all to feel more fulfilled, happier and healthier.

In an ongoing quest to discover what makes people happy and healthy, experts consistently find that the same factors contribute to our mental and physical wellbeing. These include spending time outdoors and in nature; having close, meaningful relationships and enjoying shared experiences with family and friends; having a sense of purpose and belonging, continuing to learn and giving back to the community.

So, how do we go about building this into our busy everyday lives? In the following four chapters you'll find more than 60 suggestions to inspire you to try some new experiences or do the things you usually do but with different eyes. Think of it as a handbook for health and happiness that you can dip in and out of for inspiration on how to spend your precious free time in a way that will also enhance your wellbeing. Many of the activities can be experienced in and around National Trust places. Or you can try them out at home, in your back garden, on your walk to work or on holiday. Alone or with family or friends. But first, a little more on how it works and why it matters.

LIVING WITH THE SEASONS

The changing of the seasons has a significant effect on our minds and bodies, from metabolism to brain function and mood. At least one in 50 people in the UK suffer from SAD (Seasonal Affective Disorder) where a lack of daylight causes depressive symptoms during the winter months. Many more of us will experience a milder but still

'The world is full of magic things, patiently waiting for our senses to grow sharper.'

W. B. Yeats

noticeable shift in mood, energy levels and appetite as the seasons change. It's easy to forget now we live in houses with light and warmth available at the flick of a switch and shop in supermarkets where we can buy summer fruits and vegetables all year round, but we are as connected to nature as animals and plants. Making more of a conscious effort to live with the seasons by getting outdoors more, eating seasonally and adjusting our routine to the changing weather will help us to feel more in harmony with the environment and lead to greater feelings of contentment.

THE GREEN CURE

Nature is right here all around us and we only need to get outdoors and engage our senses to experience the healing benefits of the natural world. Researchers at the University of East Anglia collected data from over 140 studies in 20 countries and concluded that spending time in green space provides 'diverse and significant health benefits'. These include a reduced risk of cardiovascular disease and diabetes, lowering of pulse, blood pressure and cortisol (stress hormone) levels, and increased sleep duration. In Japan, *shirin-yoku* or 'forest bathing' was introduced in the 1980s and what is essentially spending time among trees in woodland or parks (no bathing suit required!) has become an integral part of their national health programme. There are so many ways in which we can tap into this great natural healer that are free and available to everybody, no matter where you live – whether in the city or the countryside. From going for a walk to tending a veg patch, sketching a flower or listening to birdsong, if we switch off autopilot and tune into our environment, we can quickly start to feel the benefits.

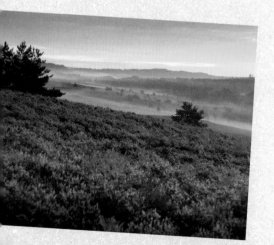

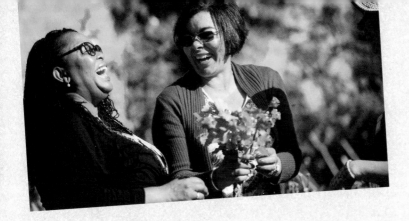

WHY PEOPLE MATTER

In our increasingly busy lives where we can communicate quickly and easily with a short text or simple 'like', it's easy to slip out of the habit of meeting up with people. Many of us unconsciously neglect our 'real-life' relationships. Yet there is extensive evidence to suggest that having close, positive communications with family and friends helps us to live longer and happier lives. One of the longest-ever-running studies into human development, The Harvard Study of Adult Development, found that over wealth, success or status, it was how happy people were in their relationships that had the greatest influence on future health and happiness. A study at Nottingham Trent University showed that belonging to a social group of people who share our passions, values and interests increases happiness levels by nine per cent for every group you join. The increasing number of clubs and activities available has made it a lot easier to foster these health-giving relationships. Whether it's running, reading, baking or painting, doing something that you enjoy with like-minded people is like a prescription for health and happiness.

NEVER STOP LEARNING

If we can be sociable while also keeping our brains busy by learning some new skills, even better. Research shows that if as adults we continue to learn in the way that we do as children we can slow the decline in cognitive function that we often notice as we hit middle age and beyond. Rather than concentrating on what we know or are good at (specialised learning), if we challenge ourselves with more varied and unfamiliar activities (broad learning), we are less likely to experience forgetfulness and loss of mental sharpness. So, if you're a very active person, try something that requires calm concentration like painting. If you prefer to work on your own, do a team activity like bushcraft or conservation. If you're worried about failing, try to unleash that inner child who faced new challenges every day, and keep on trying.

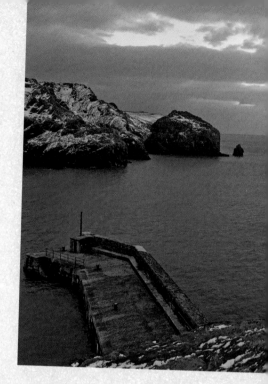

GIVING BACK

Being kind and helping others has been proven to have a positive effect on our own mental health and wellbeing. According to The Mental Health Foundation, people who are altruistic feel a sense of purpose and belonging, have a more positive outlook and higher self-esteem. Helping others doesn't have to be time-consuming or cost money. Small random acts of kindness such as offering your seat, helping an elderly person with their shopping or just telling a friend how much you appreciate them will make them feel good and you feel happier. If you have a few spare hours, volunteering or mentoring enables you to meet people while also giving something back to the community. Remember that the more you do for others, the more they'll do for you.

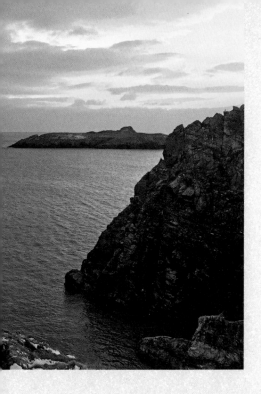

LIVE WELL ALL YEAR

The book is divided into four chapters to guide you through the year and highlight the best of spring, summer, autumn and winter. Of course, many of the ideas can be tried at any time of year and you will do things as and when they feel right for you. Some ideas will naturally appeal to you more than others but try to do a few that don't instantly leap off the page or even feel a bit too obvious upon first impression. Why? Because the brain responds well to the unexpected and stepping out of our comfort zone helps to challenge our fears and preconceptions of what we can and can't do or do and don't like. Some of the things you might do already, yet by doing them with more awareness you may notice a different and more positive outcome. For example, next time you go out for a walk you could try a different route, take off your shoes and paddle in a stream or stop and sit for a while and look up at the clouds. Perhaps you'll feel inspired to send a card or pick up the phone and arrange to meet someone you haven't heard from in a while.

You don't need to invest a lot of time or money to improve your wellbeing nor venture far to have an adventure. A breath of fresh air can be enough to change the course of a day.

For many of the activities, we have included some ideas of spots around the National Trust where you can enjoy them. But there are many more places we couldn't squeeze in. For more information on the activities and where you can enjoy them near you, visit **nationaltrust.org.uk/ breath-of-fresh-air**

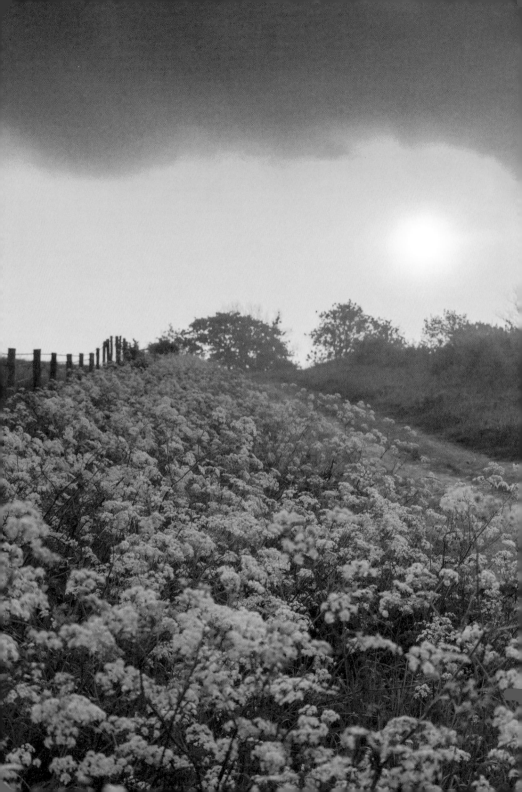

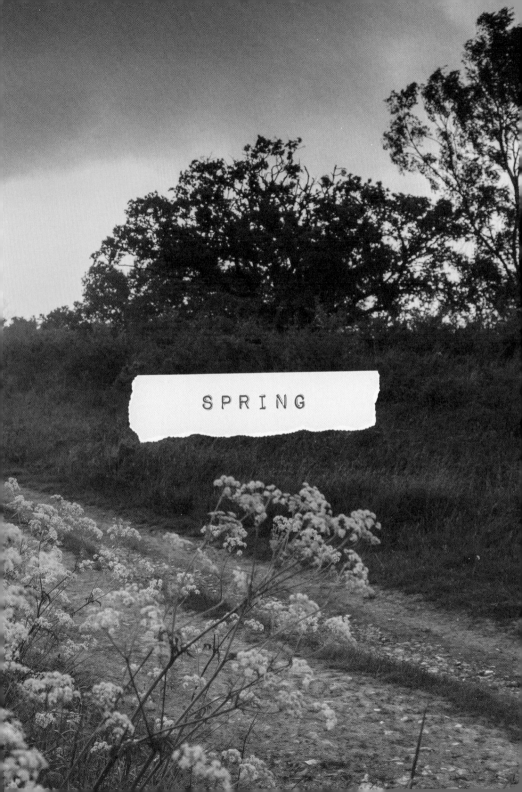

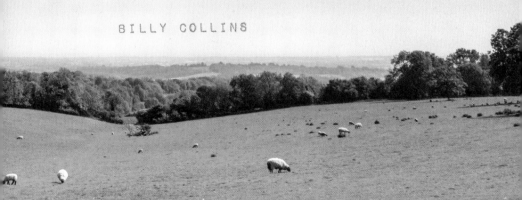

Today

If ever there were a spring day so perfect,
so uplifted by a warm intermittent breeze

that it made you want to throw
open all the windows in the house

and unlatch the door to the canary's cage,
indeed, rip the little door from its jamb,

a day when the cool brick paths
and the garden bursting with peonies

seemed so etched in sunlight
that you felt like taking

a hammer to the glass paperweight
on the living room end table,

releasing the inhabitants
from their snow-covered cottage

so they could walk out,
holding hands and squinting

into this larger dome of blue and white,
well, today is just that kind of day.

BILLY COLLINS

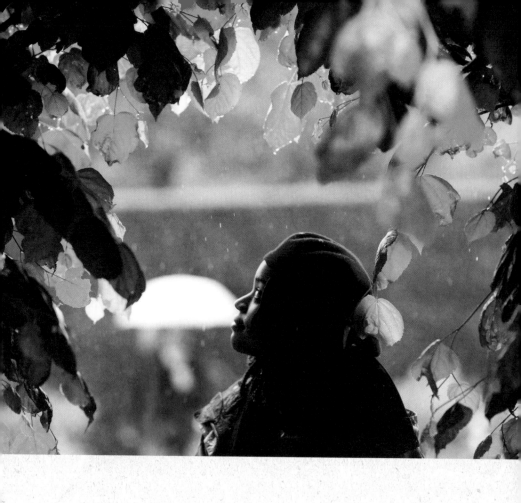

WEATHER
the WEATHER

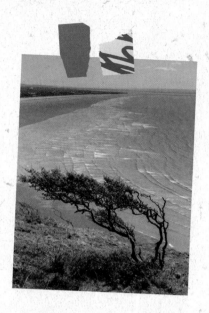

Spring has always flung unpredictable weather our way. We expect March to come 'in like a lion and out like a lamb' and nod our heads wisely if April dumps snow on us, for it is, as T. S. Eliot famously wrote, 'the cruellest month'. If you live in Britain you may as well learn to embrace the changing climate and get outdoors whatever the weather. Cold rain can feel as good against the face as warm sunshine and, as the saying goes, 'bad weather always looks worse from the window'.

SMELL THE RAIN

Ever noticed the pleasant earthy smell that comes after rainfall? It's actually got a name – petrichor – and is caused by a molecule in the soil called geosmin that is produced when water droplets land on the dry earth. Humans are particularly sensitive to the scent of geosmin, which we find calming, so much so that it's used as an ingredient in perfumes. Rain also makes the air fresher and cleaner as raindrops attract particles of pollutants, clearing the air. If you're out walking during or just after rainfall take some big deep breaths, in through the nose and out through the mouth. If there's been a thunderstorm, you should notice a significant improvement in air quality and a fresh, clean scent of ozone.

15

INHALING SUNSHINE

Make the most of the restorative powers of the sun with this easy yoga sequence, which is lovely done sitting outside or by a window on a warm day with the sun shining on your body. Sun breaths are often performed at the beginning or end of yoga practice to ease out the shoulders, back, neck and arms.

FIND A COMFORTABLE WAY TO SIT, EITHER CROSS-LEGGED OR KNEELING, SITTING ON A BLOCK IF IT HELPS YOU TO KEEP A STRAIGHT BACK.

CLOSE YOUR EYES AND INHALE, SLOWLY SWEEPING THE ARMS OUT TO THE SIDE AND UP ABOVE YOUR HEAD, BRINGING YOUR PALMS TOGETHER ABOVE YOUR HEAD.

EXHALE, BRINGING THE HANDS DOWN IN FRONT OF THE BODY INTO PRAYER POSITION.

REPEAT THREE MORE TIMES.

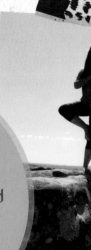

Practising yoga not only improves strength, flexibility and posture – it makes you feel happier and calmer, and improves concentration

LET THE WIND BLOW

Of all the weather systems wind can be the most unsettling. Lying in bed hearing the trees swaying and the wind whistling, you can't help but feel the greatness of nature. Hippocrates believed that the wind determined our health depending on which direction it was blowing and, in Chinese medicine, wind in the body reflects wind in nature, generating movement and bringing sudden change. All that aside, windy weather can be truly invigorating. A bracing walk on the beach or a cycle ride with the wind in your hair is energising, uplifting, rosy-cheek-inducing and really good fun, as long as you're careful of course.

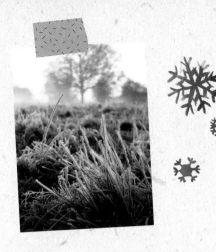

A FROSTY MORNING

A spring frost takes us all by surprise, particularly as it often follows a warm, sunny day. New-born lambs look bewildered at the sudden appearance of cold, white crystals underfoot and spring flowers bow their heads until temperatures rise again. Gardeners will be wise to leave tender bedding plants in the greenhouse or potting shed until the danger of frosts has passed, usually late May in the UK. A frosty morning is a beautiful sight and a morning walk will set you up nicely for the day ahead. Just remember to wear layers as you'll soon be peeling them off again.

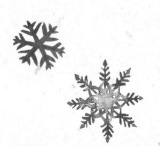

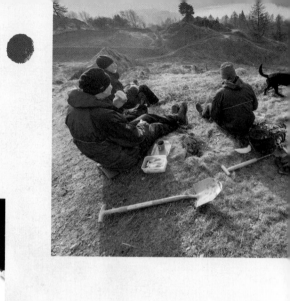

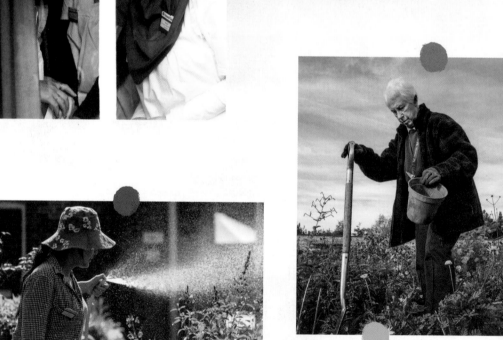

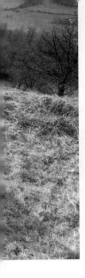

GIVE BACK AND FEEL GREAT

Volunteering not only helps get a job done but it brings you together with people in your community and can give you the opportunity to spend more time in a place that you love. The National Trust has over 500 different volunteering roles from beach cleaning to marshalling runs and greeting visitors. People who volunteer say they feel happier, less stressed and more confident. What are you waiting for?

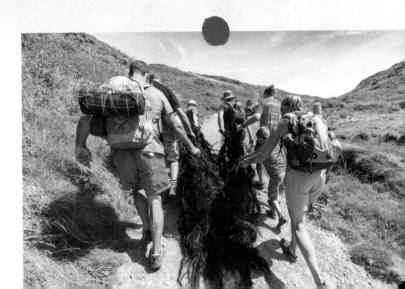

Walk with a dog

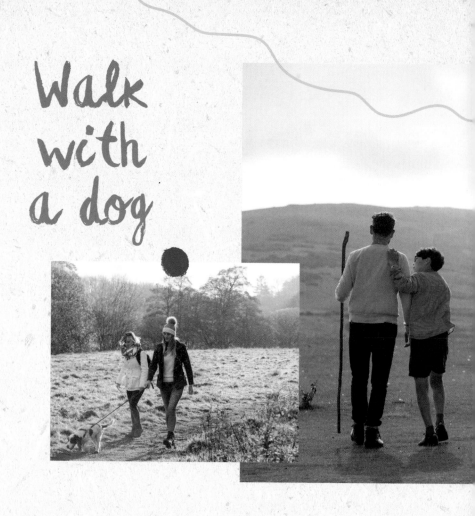

A dog will get you outdoors even on the most miserable of days and when they bound on ahead looking back at you with unfettered gratitude and happiness it can't fail to make you smile. There's much evidence showing the wellbeing benefits of dog ownership, from the obvious (exercise, companionship) to the more subtle (pets enable social interaction and reduce anxiety). We can't all own a dog, but we can borrow one. Offer to help out a friend or neighbour by taking their dog for a walk or pet-sitting while they're away. Or register with borrowmydoggy.com

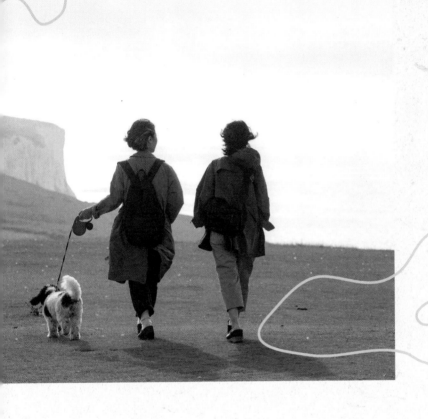

to find dog owners near you in need of a helping hand. There are many dog-friendly walks in National Trust locations, from wide sandy beaches (Studland Bay, Dorset; Dunwich Heath, Suffolk; Stackpole, Pembrokeshire) to acres of park and woodland (Morden Hall Park, London; Clumber Park, Nottinghamshire). You could join an organised dog walk (Bodnant Garden, Conwy) and enjoy a cuppa in one of the Trust's dog-friendly cafés (Gibside, Tyne & Wear). Just check the website first to ensure you pick the best spot for you and your four-legged companion.

EMBRACE CHANGE

The changing of seasons is a great opportunity to reflect on the passing of time and new beginnings. Change is something many of us find difficult to come to terms with, yet life is a natural and inevitable series of changes. Observing transformations in nature can help us to accept that everything in life is in flux and encourage us to let things flow naturally forward rather than resist it, which can lead to unhappiness.

This short meditation is to be done outside and will help you feel calmer and more accepting of any changes that are taking place in your life, however big or small. Find a quiet spot to sit outside for a while, making sure you're comfortable. Sit with your eyes open and ask yourself the following:

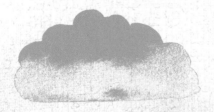

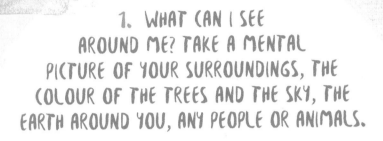

1. WHAT CAN I SEE
AROUND ME? TAKE A MENTAL
PICTURE OF YOUR SURROUNDINGS, THE
COLOUR OF THE TREES AND THE SKY, THE
EARTH AROUND YOU, ANY PEOPLE OR ANIMALS.

2. WHAT HAPPENS AS I SIT? DO THE TREES MOVE
IN THE WIND, DO ANY LEAVES FALL OR BRANCHES
CREAK? DO THE CLOUDS MOVE? DOES THE LIGHT
CHANGE? WHAT ARE THE MOVEMENTS
OF THE PEOPLE AND ANIMALS I CAN SEE?

After 10 or 15 minutes stop and think about
how the picture now differs from when
you first sat down.

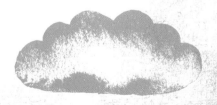

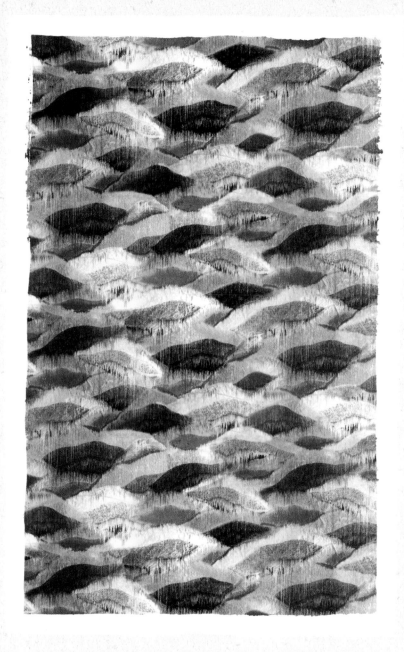

24

Turn, turn, my wheel! All things must change
To something new, to something strange;
Nothing that is can pause or stay;
The moon will wax, the moon will wane,
The mist and cloud will turn to rain,
The rain to mist and cloud again,
To-morrow be to-day.

From *Kéramos*,
Henry Wadsworth Longfellow

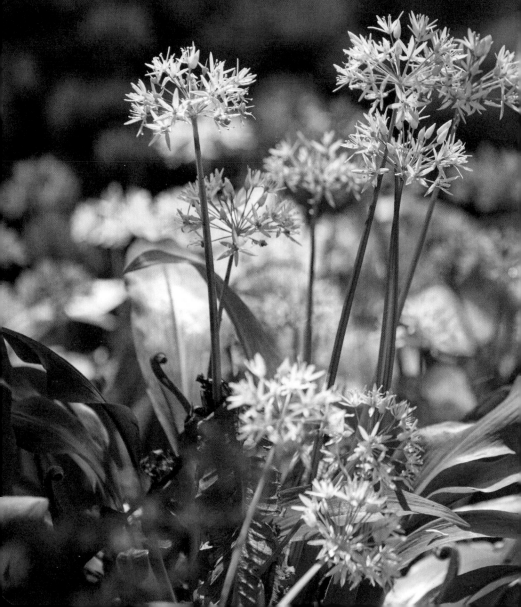

FORAGE
FOR EDIBLE
PLANTS

In the spring months our woodlands and hedgerows come to life with edible plants and flowers, and there's something so satisfying about walking home clutching hand-picked ingredients for lunch. Wild garlic grows throughout spring at many National Trust places including the ancient woodland of Smallcombe Wood just above the Bath Skyline walk, Ilam Park in Derbyshire and Erddig, Wrexham. Picking is encouraged, and in some locations, visitors are offered brown paper bags at the entrance but it's a good idea to pack a bag for your harvest. Look for young nettles, too, in early spring (just make sure you wear rubber gloves when picking). Both wild garlic and nettles make tasty and nutritious additions to soups, salads and omelettes. The young leaves and flowers of the hawthorn are edible and have a pleasant nutty taste, and a sprinkling of wild flower petals such as sweet violet and dandelion make a salad look pretty and unusual.

There are important guidelines when foraging: always cut from the base rather than pulling up the bulb or roots, take a little from plentiful areas and leave enough behind for wildlife and other foragers, taking care not to trample over plants. And never pick fungi without the company of an expert. A foraging walk is the best way to get started and a very enjoyable way to pass a few hours. Check out the National Trust website for courses near you.

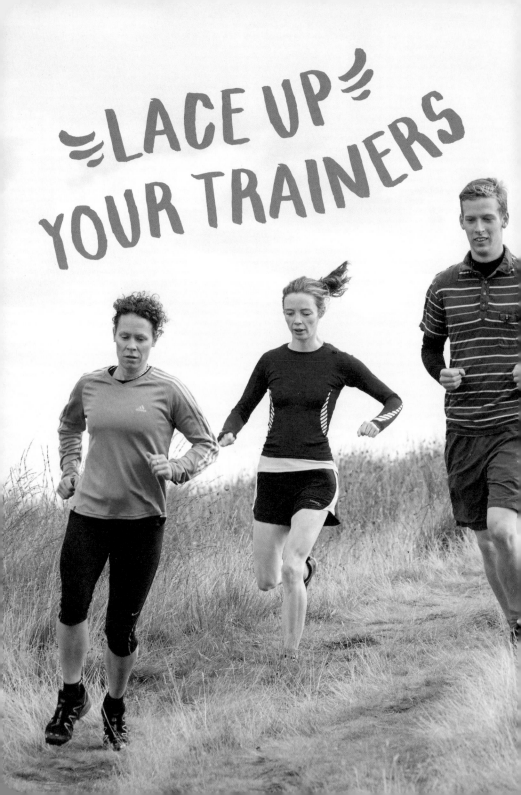

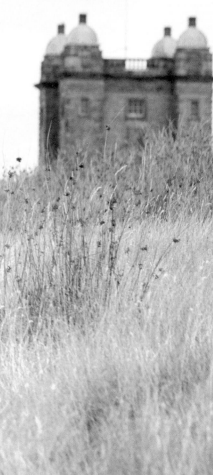

It's free, you can do it almost anywhere, it's a brilliant cardiovascular workout and it makes you feel happy. We're talking about running of course. Whether you're going on a gentle Sunday morning jog or training for an event, the National Trust has acres of land to explore where you can run at your own pace in natural surroundings away from traffic and pollution, and on terrain that's less stressful on the joints than pavements. If you want to join up with others look out for the parkrun events that take place every Saturday morning in over 20 National Trust locations. These are truly family-friendly affairs for all ages and abilities, with dogs welcome at many locations. The Trust10 trail runs are monthly 10k events, but if you prefer to go alone there are mapped-out Ranger Runs for varying levels available to print out on the National Trust website. Running is an exhilarating way to explore a new area and enjoy a bit of wildlife-spotting on the go. You could even do your bit for the environment and try a spot of plogging – that's jogging while picking up litter.

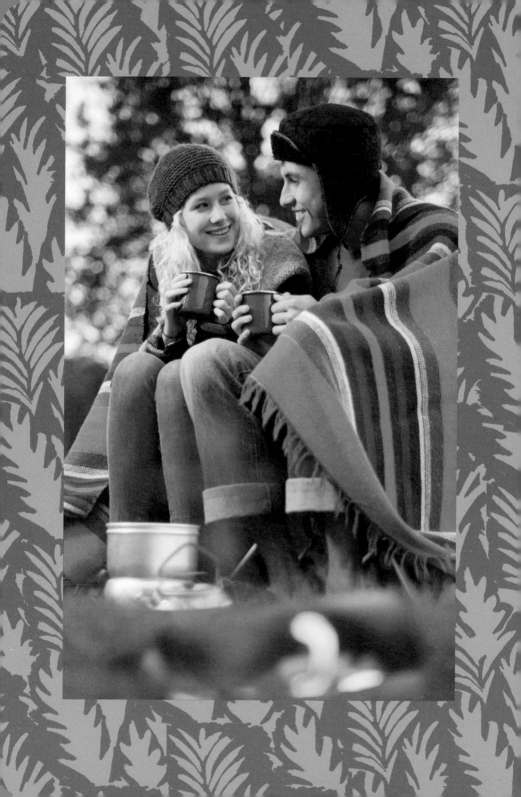

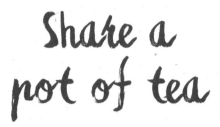

Share a pot of tea

A chat with a friend over a cup of tea is as good for you as an afternoon in a spa. Interacting with our friends brings numerous health benefits from lowering blood pressure and cortisol levels (stress hormones) to boosting self-esteem and happiness. Share a pot of good tea and a slice of fluffy sponge cake somewhere that makes you happy, with someone that makes you smile, and never feel guilty about taking a tea break.

Get your hands dirty

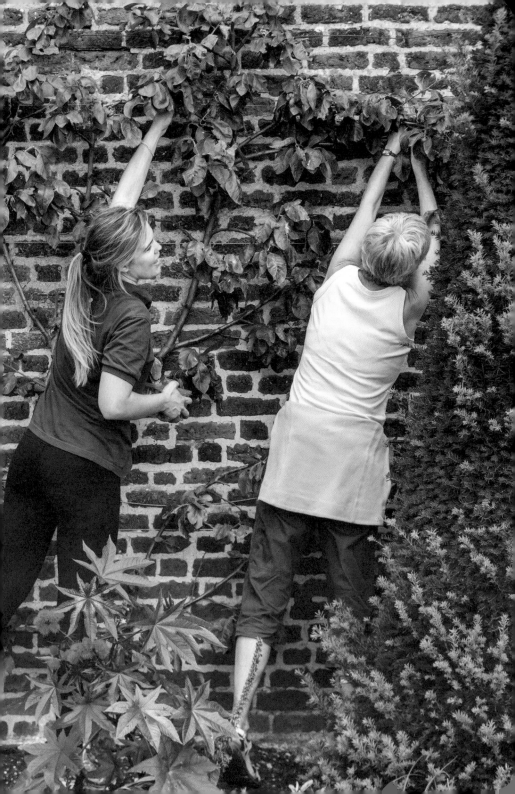

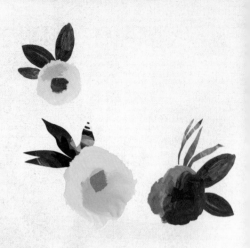

Plant a window box, pot some herbs or do a spot of weeding and, as well as basking in the rewards of your labour, you'll boost your health in the process. The reason many gardeners seem so content might not just be the fresh air and physical activity (although that definitely helps). Soil contains microbes that have been proven to boost our immunity and mental health when we come into contact with them, either on our skin or by digesting them. Don't be afraid to get your hands dirty; see soil down your nails as a sign you're looking after your health and, where possible, why not try to grow some of what you eat (home-grown lettuce leaves and herbs are an easy way to get an instant dose of health-boosting microbes)? If you don't have a garden or would like to get your hands on something a little different, there are volunteering opportunities in some very exciting outdoor places where you can get involved in planting and pruning or planning and tending allotments. Garden volunteers get to develop and hone their skills, work as part of a team and share their knowledge with visitors either in passing conversation or as a garden guide.

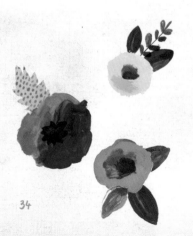

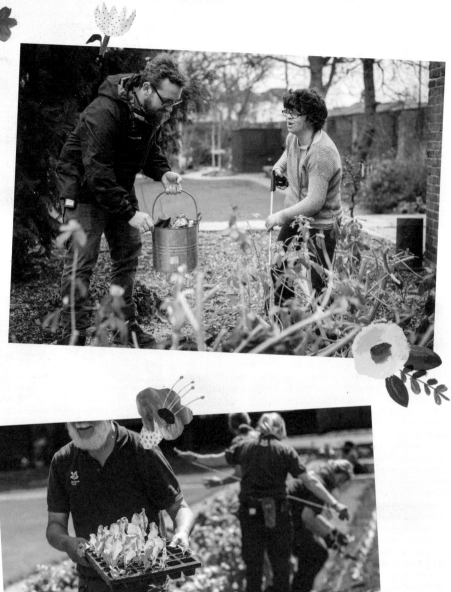

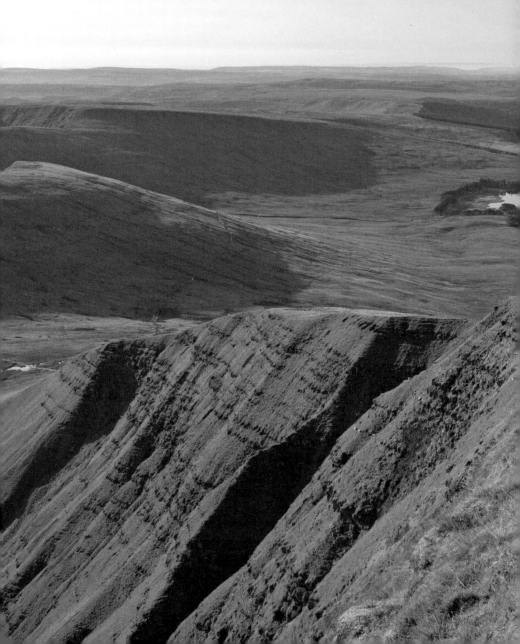

'NOT ALL THOSE WHO

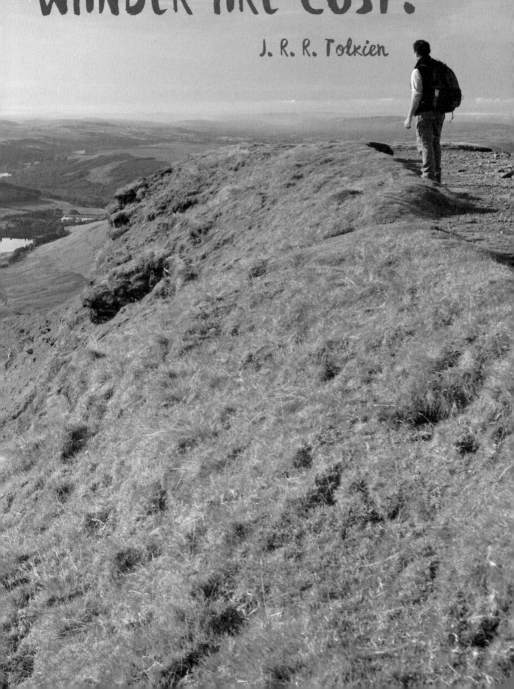

WANDER ARE LOST.'

J. R. R. Tolkien

GET A LITTLE LOST

How many times do you switch on Google Maps when really you know the way? Relying on maps makes us less observant and curious, so when you can afford to take a little longer and risk getting a little lost it can be fun to switch your phone off or put away the guide and just let yourself wander. Try this when you're out walking in a pair or as a group and notice how simply changing your route alters your perspective and see if it leads to any unexpected discoveries (even if it's only that you did know the way after all).

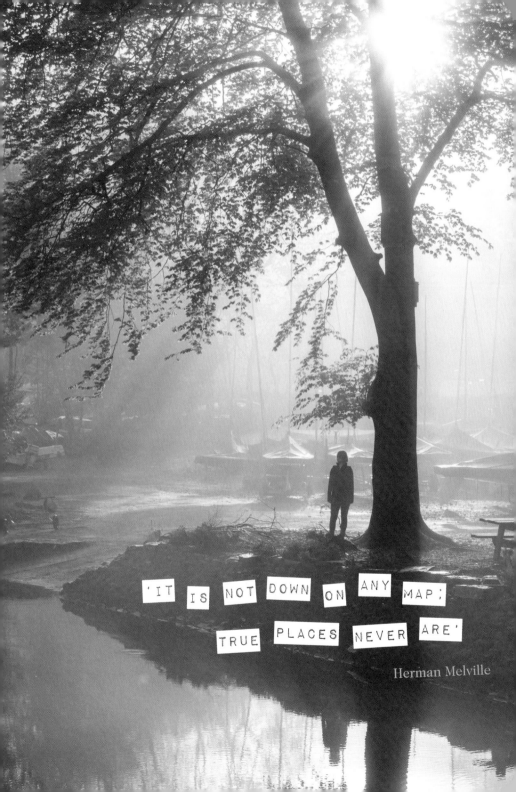

'IT IS NOT DOWN ON ANY MAP;
TRUE PLACES NEVER ARE'

Herman Melville

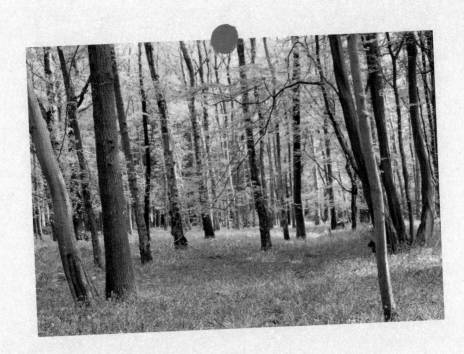

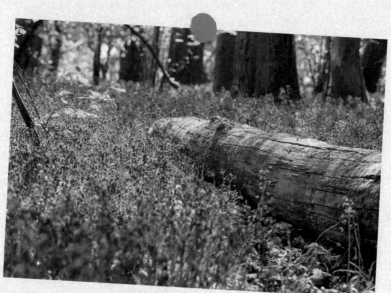

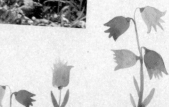

It's impossible not to feel uplifted by the sight of a woodland carpeted in bluebells. One of the prettiest wild flowers, with its distinctive shape and vivid shades of blue and violet, it has stopped many a walker in their tracks. Although half of the world's bluebell population is found in the UK, the English bluebell is becoming rarer to spot.

trample and never to pick, and you'll capture their sweet, strong scent. The Spanish variety and hybrids are what you usually see in gardens and are a paler blue with flowers all around the stem and no scent. Find bluebells galore at Blickling Estate in Norfolk, Sheffield Park and Garden, East Sussex, Coughton Court, Warwickshire and Hardcastle Crags, West

WANDER THROUGH A BLUEBELL WOOD

They're usually found in woodland and shady areas, and the flowers, which are only on one side of the stem, have a narrow, straight-sided bell with parallel sides and curled edges. Bend over the flowers, taking care not to

Yorkshire (or find your nearest bluebell wood on the National Trust website). When you strike blue, why not take a photo and save it as your screensaver so you can recapture that spring feeling on grey days?

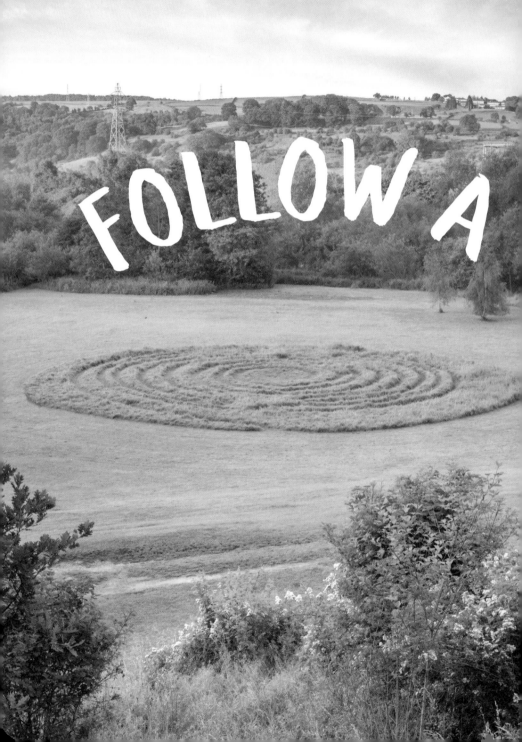

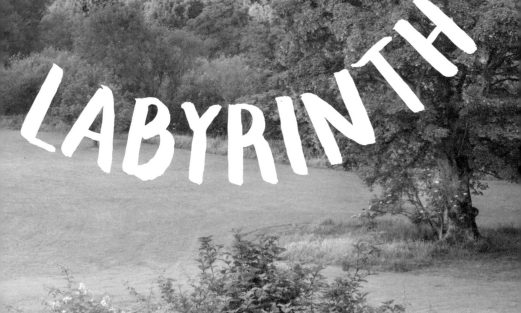

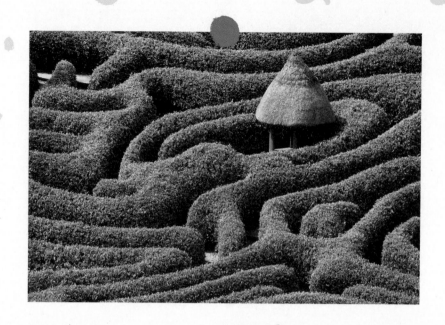

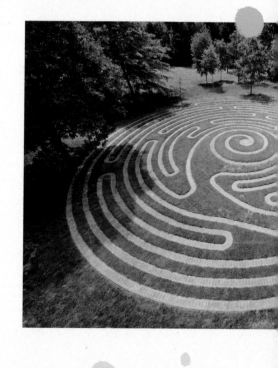

Walking through the winding paths of a maze or labyrinth is a mesmerising activity whatever your age. From the 17th-century labyrinth at Lyveden in Northamptonshire and the recently restored 18th-century labyrinth at Stowe in Buckinghamshire to intricate garden mazes, such as Glendurgan Garden, Cornwall, you can let your mind unwind as you follow the pathways marked out with stones, trees, hedges, long grass or flowering shrubs. From medieval times and earlier, walking a labyrinth would have symbolised the pilgrimage through life, offering a time to reflect and pray. Explore slowly and mindfully, taking off your shoes if you fancy it, and when you get to the middle make sure to sit or stand and pause for a while before you set off back again. In case you were wondering what the difference is, a labyrinth has one single path leading clockwise into the centre, while a maze has multiple entrances and exits, and deliberately confusing paths and dead ends.

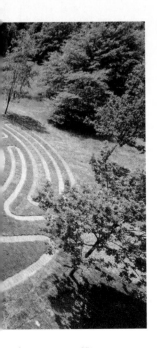

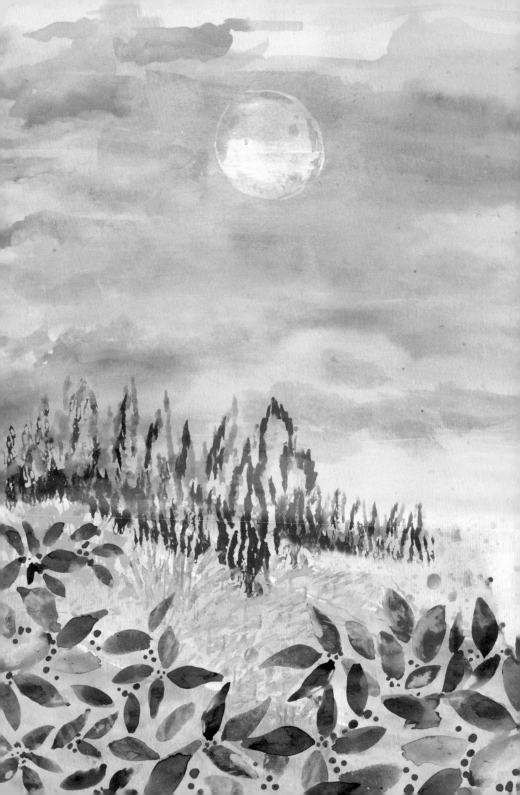

'Sunshine is delicious,
rain is refreshing,
wind braces us up,
snow is exhilarating;
there is really no such
thing as bad weather,
only different kinds of
good weather.' John Ruskin

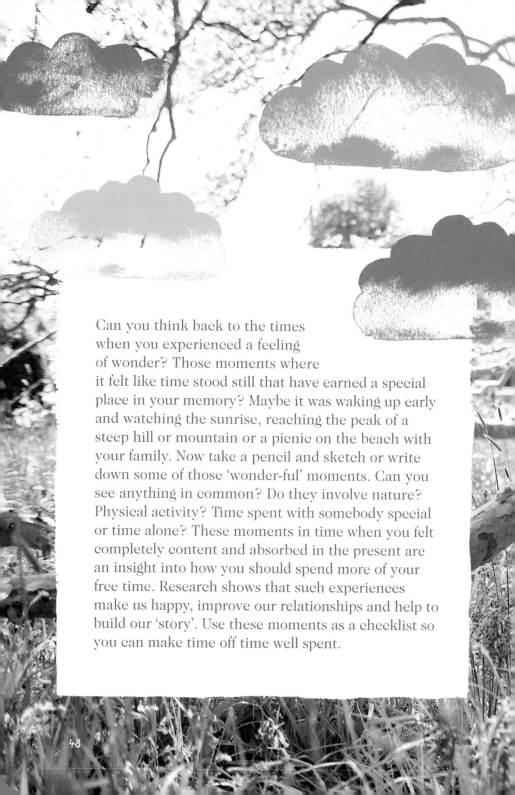

Can you think back to the times
when you experienced a feeling
of wonder? Those moments where
it felt like time stood still that have earned a special
place in your memory? Maybe it was waking up early
and watching the sunrise, reaching the peak of a
steep hill or mountain or a picnic on the beach with
your family. Now take a pencil and sketch or write
down some of those 'wonder-ful' moments. Can you
see anything in common? Do they involve nature?
Physical activity? Time spent with somebody special
or time alone? These moments in time when you felt
completely content and absorbed in the present are
an insight into how you should spend more of your
free time. Research shows that such experiences
make us happy, improve our relationships and help to
build our 'story'. Use these moments as a checklist so
you can make time off time well spent.

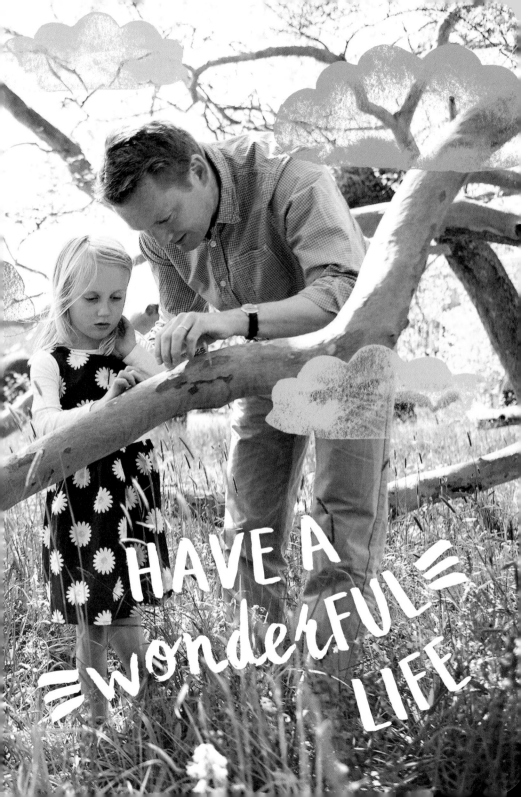

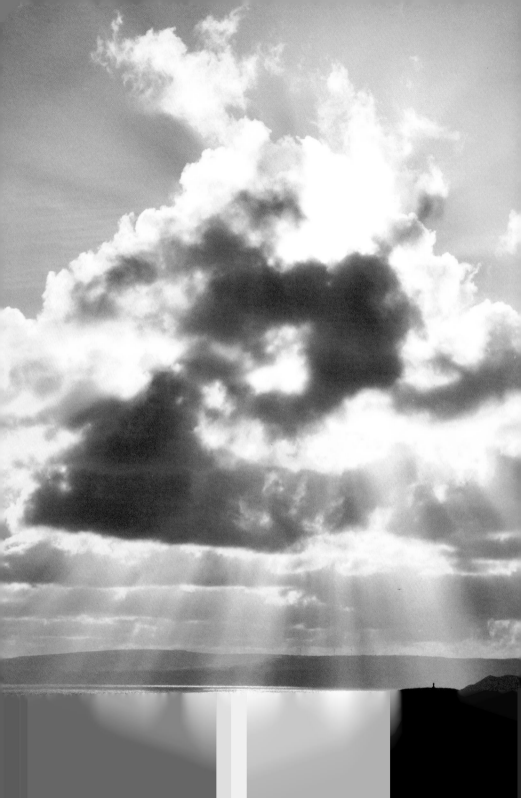

'AWARENESS IS LIKE THE SUN. WHEN IT SHINES ON THINGS, THEY ARE TRANSFORMED.'

Thich Nhat Hanh, Buddhist monk and peace activist

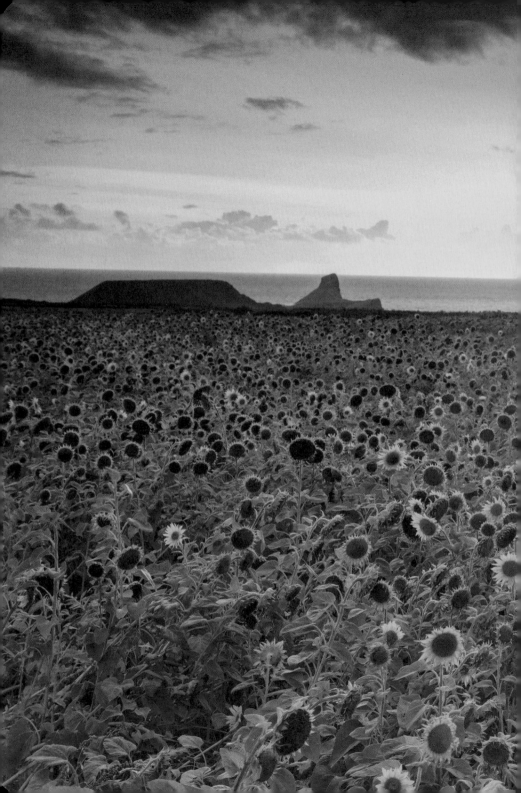

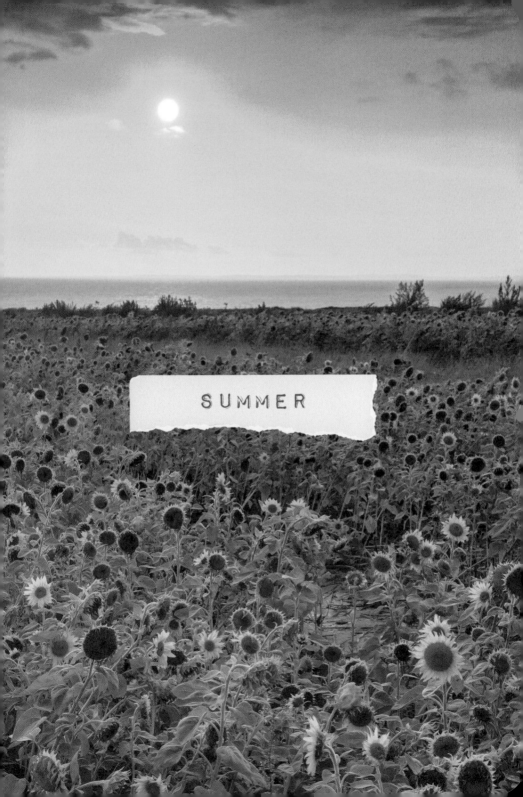

LEISURE

What is this life if, full of care,
We have no time to stand and stare –

No time to stand beneath the boughs
And stare as long as sheep or cows:

No time to see, when woods we pass,
Where squirrels hide their nuts in grass:

No time to see, in broad daylight,
Streams full of stars, like skies at night:

No time to turn at Beauty's glance,
And watch her feet, how they can dance:

No time to wait till her mouth can
Enrich that smile her eyes began?

A poor life this is if, full of care,
We have no time to stand and stare.

WILLIAM HENRY DAVIES

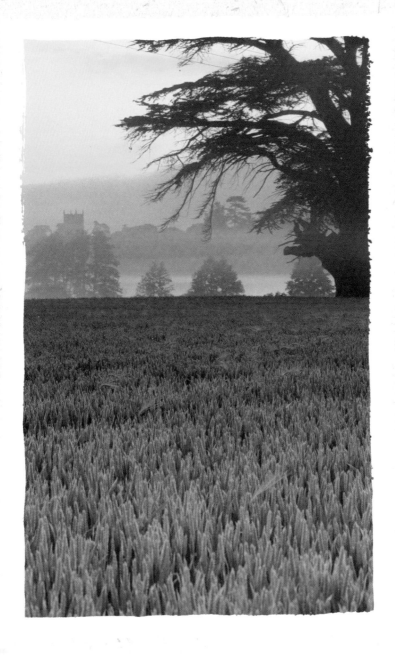

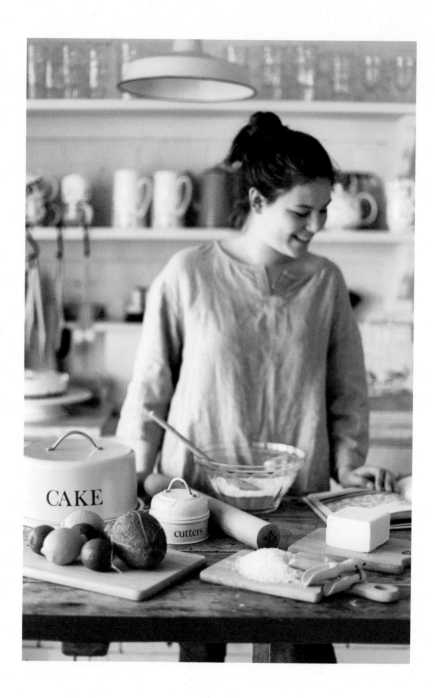

CATCH (and pass on) THE KINDNESS BUG

Kindness is contagious. Do something spontaneously thoughtful for somebody today and you'll start a ripple of kindness.

WAYS TO BE KIND

 Invite an elderly friend, family member or neighbour for an outing.

 Bake an extra tray of biscuits or cupcakes and give some away.

 Buy a small, thoughtful gift for someone, just because.

 Recommend a favourite book or film to a friend.

 Pass on a cutting that you have potted up from your favourite plant.

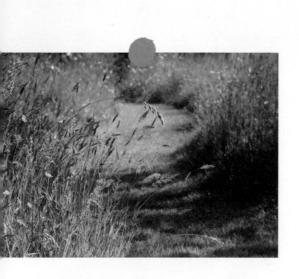

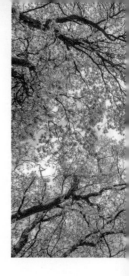

LIE IN FRESHLY MOWN GRASS

Feeling the earth beneath you is quite literally a grounding experience. Find an inviting spot in your garden, in a meadow or under a tree in the park and lie down for a while on the grass. Notice how the earth feels against your skin. Take off your shoes and place your feet on the ground, wiggling your toes a little. What does it feel like? Look around you at ground level and notice the colour and shape of the blades of grass and the detail of the petals on any wild flowers. Can you spot any insects? Watch how they move around. Lie like this for at least 10 minutes, just observing the different sights and sensations.

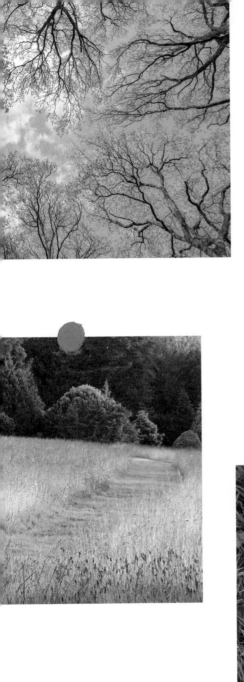

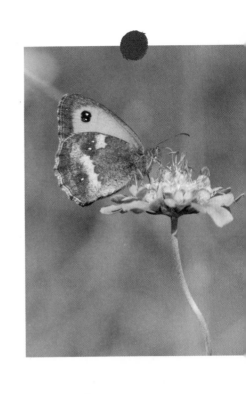

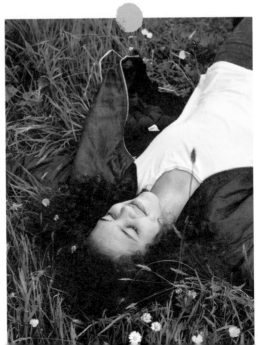

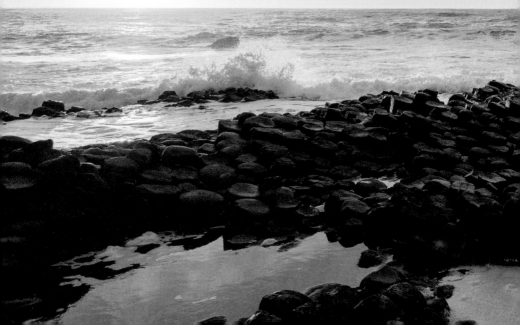

Water, EVERy

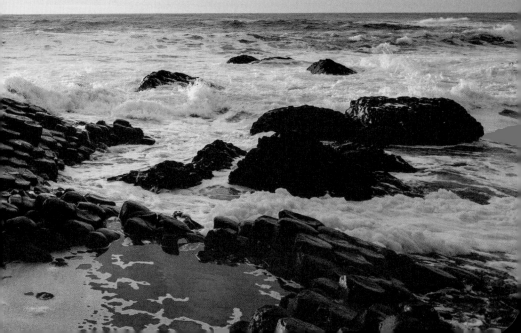

water
WHERE

Whether it's gazing at a lily pond, dipping our toes into a stream or watching waves crash onto the shore, humans are instinctively drawn to water. We listen to the sound of waterfalls for relaxation, covet bedrooms and dining tables with ocean views and visualise watery scenes in meditation sessions. And there are good scientific reasons for this – when we're around water it triggers a calm, meditative state known as 'blue mind'. Pick a watery walk to suit your mood. If you're feeling reflective you might like to sit in a serene spot such as by Fairy Lake at Ickworth in Suffolk or marvel at a natural wonder such as the dual waterfall in the bay at Hayburn Wyke, North Yorkshire. If you're in a playful mood you could rediscover your inner child while crossing the stepping stones over the River Dove in Dovedale, Derbyshire or playing Pooh sticks over Minnowburn Bridge in County Down. Whether you end up by a river, stream, lake, waterfall or ocean, try to spend a little time just watching the water and listening to the sounds around you. As your blue mind awakens let that wave of calm and contentment wash over you.

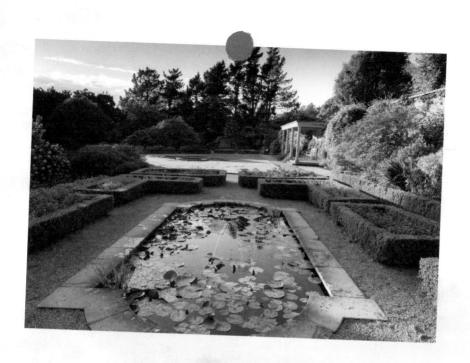

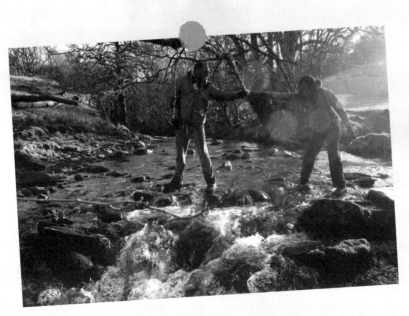

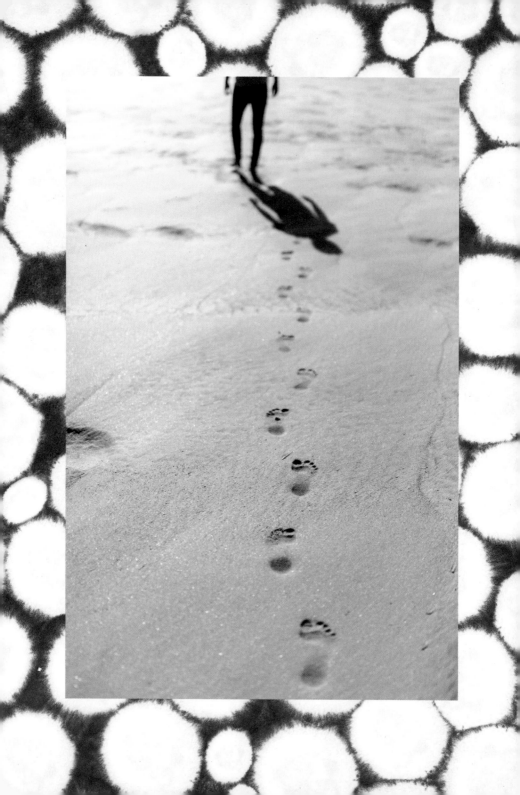

Take your shoes off

Research into the health benefits associated with connecting our bodies with the earth (known as earthing or grounding) show that it can have significant physiological and psychological benefits, from reducing pain and inflammation to improving sleep quality and reducing levels of the stress hormone, cortisol. The theory is that humans evolved in direct contact with the earth's subtle electric charge and that over time we have lost this connection, due to modern life where we live and work in buildings, drive cars and wear shoes. One of the easiest ways to feel the earth is to go barefoot. Feet function at their best when they're in their bare, natural state and the toes can flex, extend and spread. It's even better when you're outside and you feel the ground underfoot, and the feet can navigate the different terrain, as they're designed to do. Kick off your shoes in the garden, or while playing rounders. Paddle in a stream, walk along the shore, feel grass, sand and mud between your toes while giving your feet a welcome dose of the natural world.

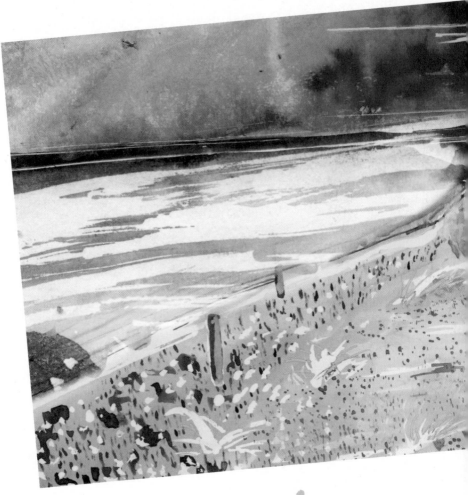

send a

postcard

Remember how much you used to enjoy receiving a postcard? Next time you're out for the day or away on holiday, send a postcard or two. Sitting down to craft a handwritten note is a mindful activity that encourages you to use your imagination, not to mention those neglected handwriting skills. It's so much more intimate than a text or social media post – just think how your card would brighten somebody's morning when it lands on their doormat.

HAVE A PICNIC IN A MEADOW

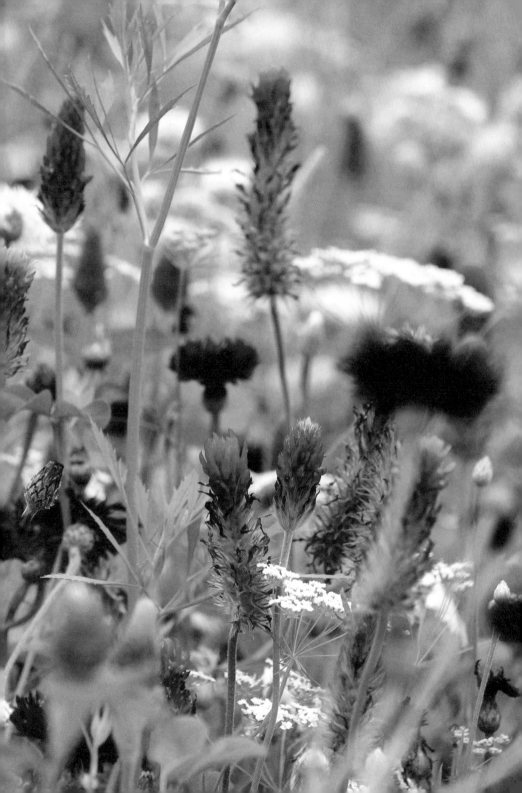

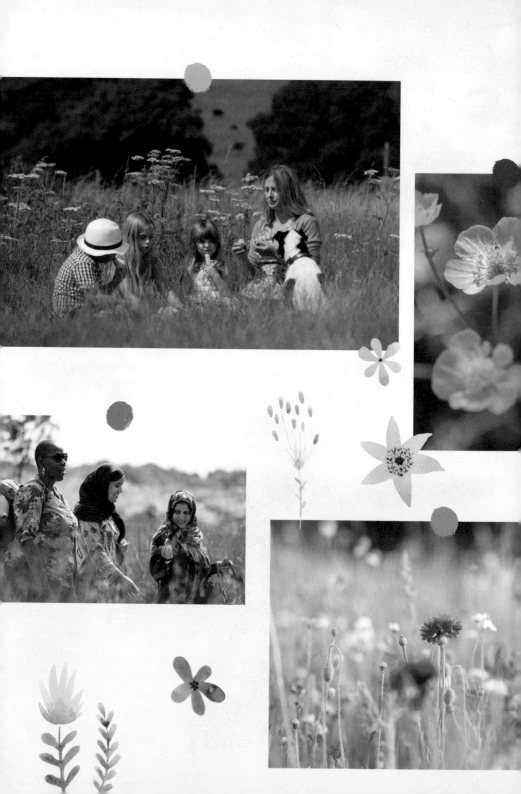

A meadow on a midsummer's day is a picnic just waiting to happen. Gather blankets, baskets, friends and family and make a date to lie among the long grass and wild flowers. This is an occasion for simple food for sharing – bowls of strawberries and cherries and a couple of good cheeses. Tear chunks from a baguette and pass it on for others to make their own sandwiches with a slice of cheese, fresh tomatoes and just-picked salad leaves. Don't forget to bring a bottle of something delicious; a light English sparkling wine would be ideal, or some cloudy lemonade. Once you've eaten, all there is to do is to sit back and relax. Lie down on the blanket and giggle and doze in the sunshine until reality calls and it's time to go home. Don't make this a once-a-year occurrence. Eating outside and sharing food with friends and family brings joy and happiness and, by picnicking, you share the shopping and the cooking and there's no clearing up to do.

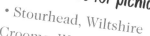

Where to find meadows made for picnics

- Stourhead, Wiltshire
- Croome, Worcestershire
- Speke Hall, Liverpool
- Winkworth Arboretum, Surrey
- Cushendun, County Antrim
- Dinefwr, Carmarthenshire
- Roseberry Topping, North Yorkshire

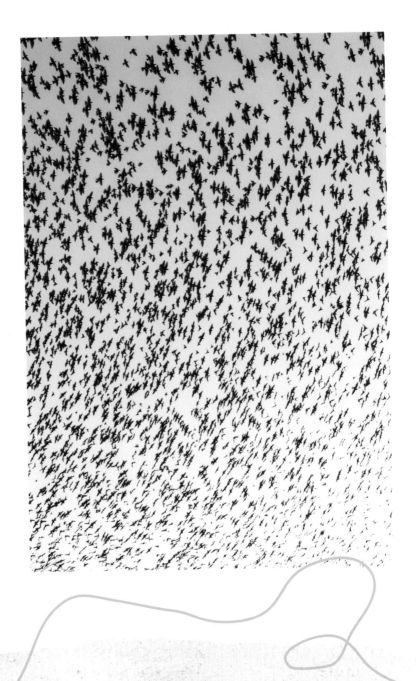

Listen carefully

Find a quiet place to sit. Listen to the sounds around you and, when something grabs your attention, try to focus on that sound in particular. Can you hear a specific birdsong? The sound of rustling in the bushes? The distant whirring of traffic or an aeroplane overhead? Somewhere that seems very quiet can actually be full of surprising sounds when you listen carefully. This creative exercise encourages you to use your senses in a different way so you think more carefully about the sounds you hear and how they make you feel.

You could write a list of sounds, doodle an image that represents the sound or use the voice-recording feature on your phone to actually record noises. It can be interesting to keep a sound diary like this and listen back to your recordings, thinking about where you were when you heard them.

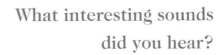

What interesting sounds
did you hear?

- _____

- _____

- _____

- _____

- _____

- _____

- _____

Al fresco arts

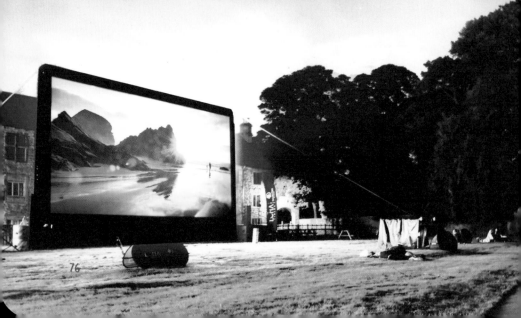

There can be few more enjoyable ways to pass a summer's evening than gathering friends to watch an outdoor film or live performance. Bring a rug, a picnic and a bottle and make the most of the long, light evenings while being entertained. Take your pick from new and classic films projected onto a big screen and many live theatre performances from Shakespeare to family favourites such as *Alice in Wonderland* and *The Secret Garden*. You can also find live music performances taking place throughout the summer, many in spectacular National Trust gardens or parkland. Don't forget to pack a blanket to ensure you stay warm and cosy as night falls.

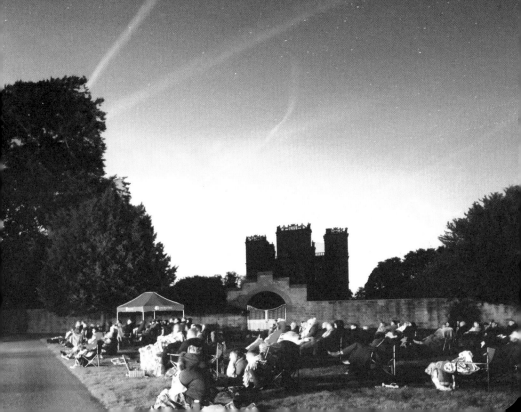

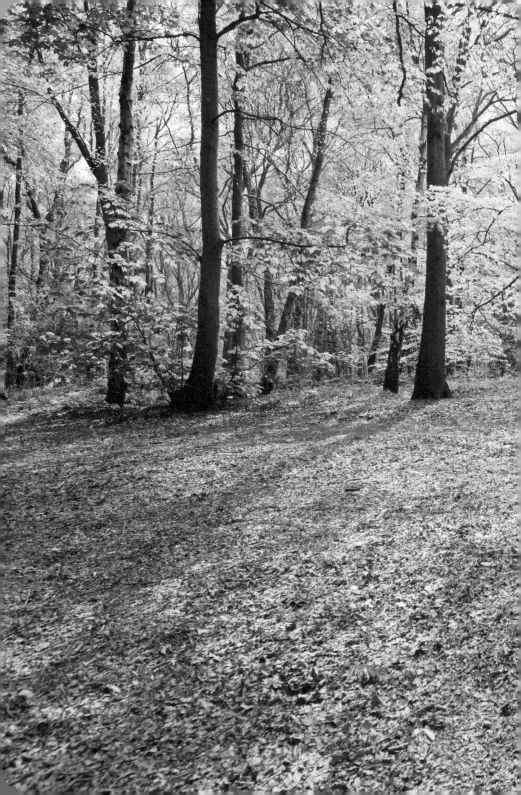

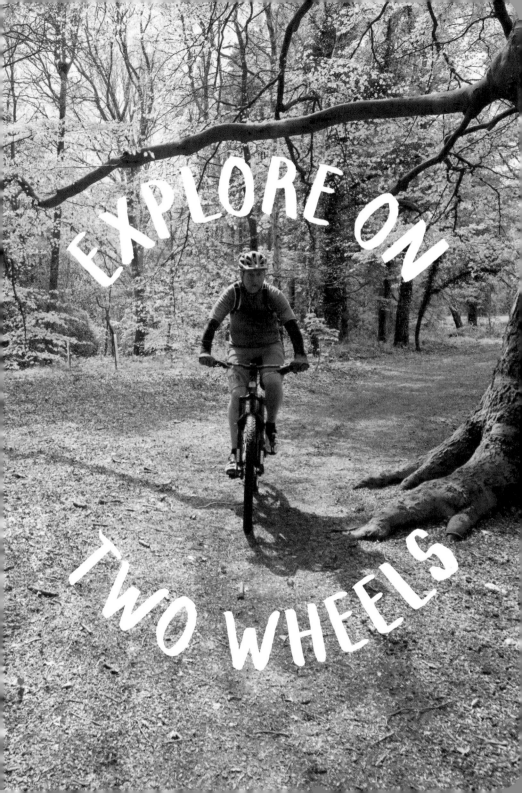

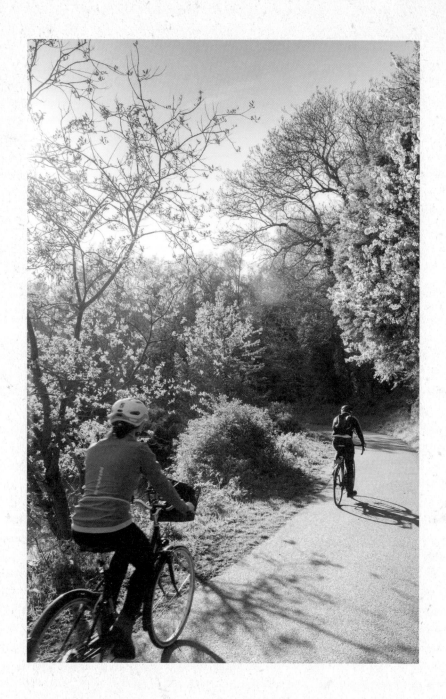

There's so much to love about cycling. The sense of freedom and childlike wonder you feel as you set off on an adventure, the connection with nature and the elements you experience as you ride, and of course the physical exertion that dissipates those stress hormones so effectively. Riding a bike requires a level of concentration that differs from walking or running. This focus helps to still the

have a bike or the means to transport yours, choose a location where you can hire one. If you're just getting back in the saddle or cycling with your young family, there are lots of easy trails to start off with, such as the four-mile off-road track at Blickling Estate in Norfolk, the old horse-drawn tramway trail at Calke Abbey, Derbyshire or Lanhydrock in Cornwall, which has off-road trails

'NOTHING COMPARES TO THE SIMPLE PLEASURE OF A BIKE RIDE.' John F. Kennedy

whirring of a busy mind and bring awareness to your body and your breath.

It doesn't matter if you're cycling alone or with others; it's your bike and your journey. One day you could be cruising along the coast and the next winding through ancient woodland or tackling a challenging hill climb. If you don't

of varying difficulty. More intrepid cyclists can find tougher trails in the Peak and Lake Districts to keep them challenged. Whether you ride all day or for an hour you'll come home feeling happy and exhilarated, having given your body and mind a workout while seeing the world from a whole new perspective.

DOZE ON A

Z
Z
Z

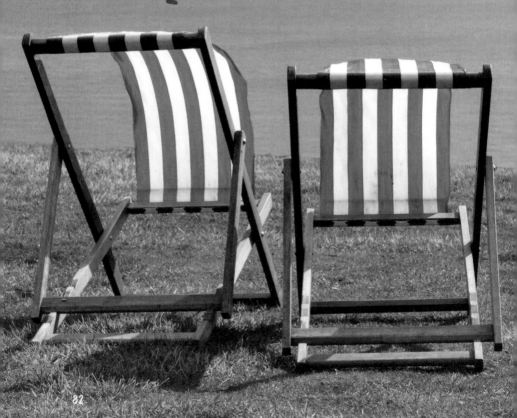

DECKCHAIR

We're all so busy being busy that doing nothing can feel awkward and uncomfortable. But we can all benefit from being a little idle from time to time and when a deckchair in the sunshine beckons it's too good an opportunity to be missed. Sit back, close your eyes and let your mind wander. See where it takes you and let yourself drift around there for a while. If you're lucky you might find yourself nodding off, and there's nothing to be ashamed of in that – a 10-minute power nap has been proven to improve alertness, mood and performance.

BE CURIOUS

THE LOST ART OF NOTICING

Too often we walk around on auto-pilot not really noticing what's around us or questioning what we see or hear. Next time you go out, take off your headphones, keep your phone in your pocket and open your eyes. It's amazing how much more you notice when you make a conscious effort to observe your surroundings.

'If you keep your eyes open
and your mind open, everything
can be interesting.'

Agnès Varda

As an exercise, draw a little map here of a route you take often – maybe a dog walk or a commute to work or walk to the local shops. Draw some of the things you remember seeing along the way. Then do the walk, but with your powers of observation switched on. What can you add to your map that you didn't notice before? You'll probably be surprised by how much you hadn't seen before. Label the drawings on your route and if you don't know what something is then find out, whether it's the history of a building or the name of a flower or bird you spotted. Keep reading, asking questions and listening, and you'll stay interested and interesting.

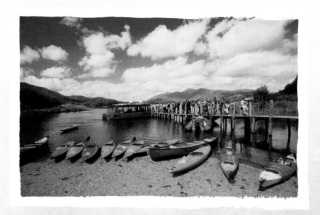

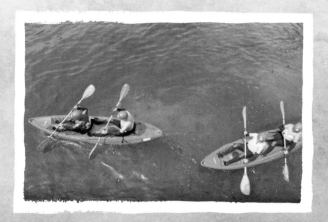

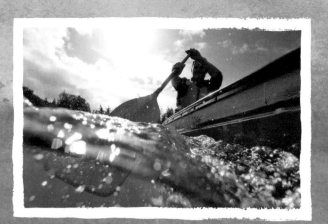

GO PADDLING

It's good to view the world from a different
perspective and when you're bobbing about on
the surface of an expanse of water you certainly
get to look at your surroundings from a fresh
angle. Canoeing or kayaking is a fun way to get
out on the water, whether you're on the sea,
a river, lake or canal, and you don't need any
experience to be able to enjoy it. Once you
get into a rhythm it's a wonderfully peaceful
and meditative activity and a great way to get
closer to wildlife, from seals at Mullion Cove in
Cornwall to birds – including the more rarely
spotted water rails at Fell Foot, Cumbria.
While paddling a canoe or kayak relaxes the
mind, your body will be working hard and you
may well have achy shoulders and abdominal
muscles on the following day. You can rent a
boat by the hour, take a guided tour or a lesson
and, if you want a different watery challenge,
stand-up paddle boarding (SUP) is increasing
in popularity. SUP helps to focus the mind and
will improve your balance and core strength;
just be prepared to get a little wet as you learn!

TURN YOUR PHONE OFF

Even if you don't consider yourself a smartphone addict, you probably spend more time on your device and are more distracted by it than you realise – the average person now spends three-and-a-half hours a day online and checks their phone 80 times a day, and it's not just teenagers that are guilty. Consider an afternoon or day of digital silence. You can phone, text or email people if you need to, but try to limit checking your device to once or twice a day and don't engage with any social media or news feeds or WhatsApp groups that aren't absolutely necessary. How does it feel to be unconnected for a little while? Do you get a strong urge to check your phone and does that feeling lessen with time? When you don't have one eye on your phone, you'll find you listen more, enjoy conversations and feel more present and engaged with your surroundings and the company you're in.

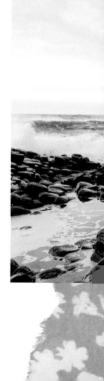

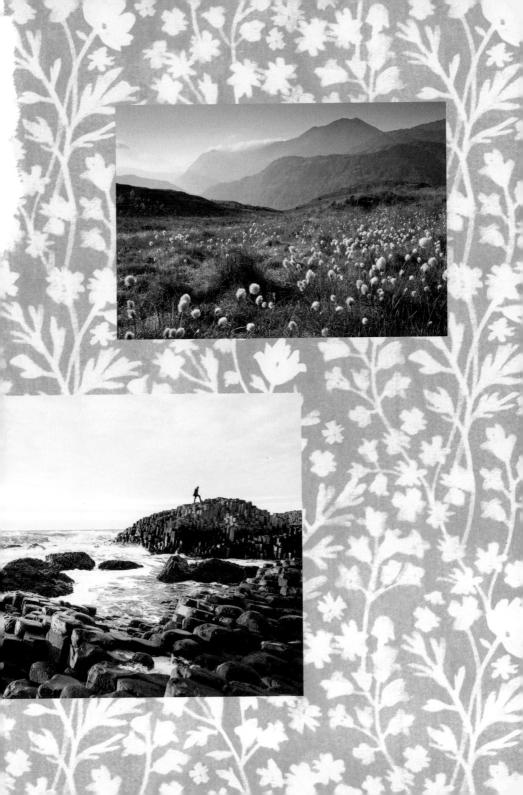

Be a mindful birdwatcher

We have a lot to gain by paying attention to and appreciating what wonderful creatures birds are and what they can offer us. Birdwatching doesn't have to mean being able to identify every bird you come across – a more meaningful way to enjoy birds is to really watch, listen and get to know the habits of a few rather than the names of a hundred. There's evidence that listening to birdsong is good for our wellbeing, leading us into a state of 'relaxed alertness' and improving our mood. And if we look out and listen for birds as we sit or walk, it leads to a greater feeling of connection with nature and our environment.

It helps to sit quietly for a while to tune into the different sights and sounds, and to encourage birds to come closer to you. This 'Sit Spot' exercise is recommended for observing wildlife. Sit or lie still for at least 20 minutes in one spot and notice what you can see and hear around you. Pick somewhere nice and quiet where you won't get disturbed, preferably close to your home so you can return to the place regularly – it might even be in your garden. Start to recognise the birds that you see there, tune into their song and observe their behaviours. Notice how their calls change as you sit and ask yourself what it might be that they're communicating. Take a guided birdwatching walk or download an app to help you to recognise and identify different birds and their language, but be warned it's a highly addictive pastime.

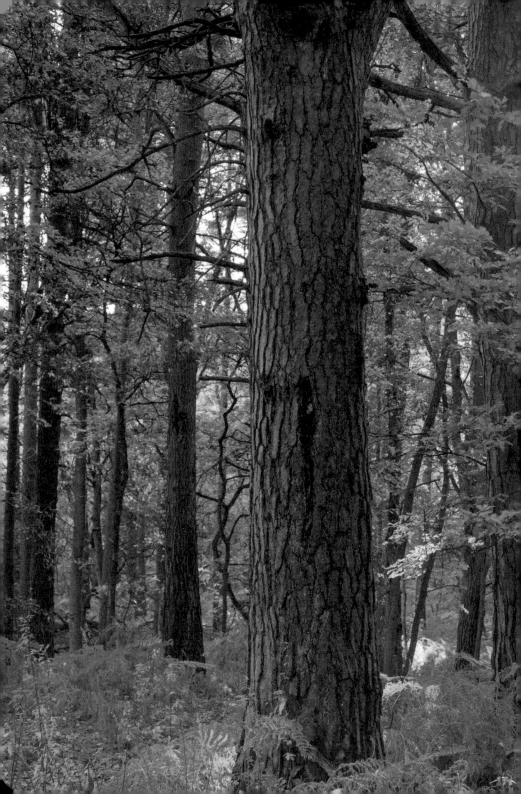

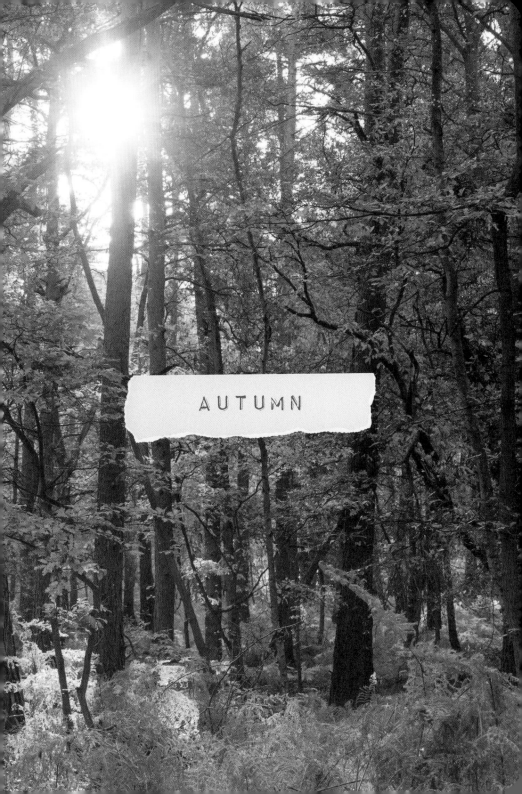

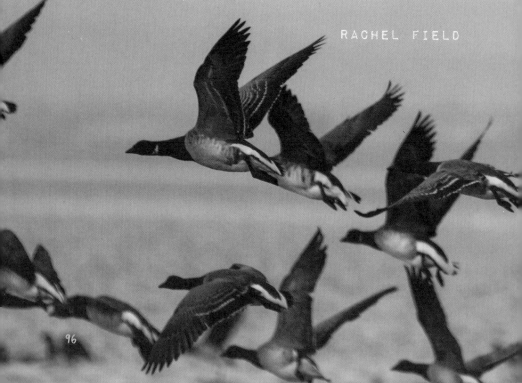

Something Told the Wild Geese

Something told the wild geese
It was time to go.
Though the fields lay golden
Something whispered,—'Snow.'
Leaves were green and stirring,
Berries, luster-glossed,
But beneath warm feathers
Something cautioned,—'Frost.'
All the sagging orchards
Steamed with amber spice,
But each wild breast stiffened
At remembered ice.
Something told the wild geese
It was time to fly,—
Summer sun was on their wings,
Winter in their cry.

RACHEL FIELD

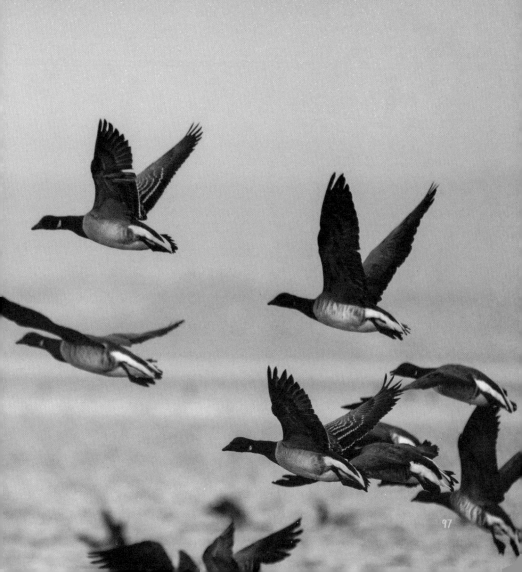

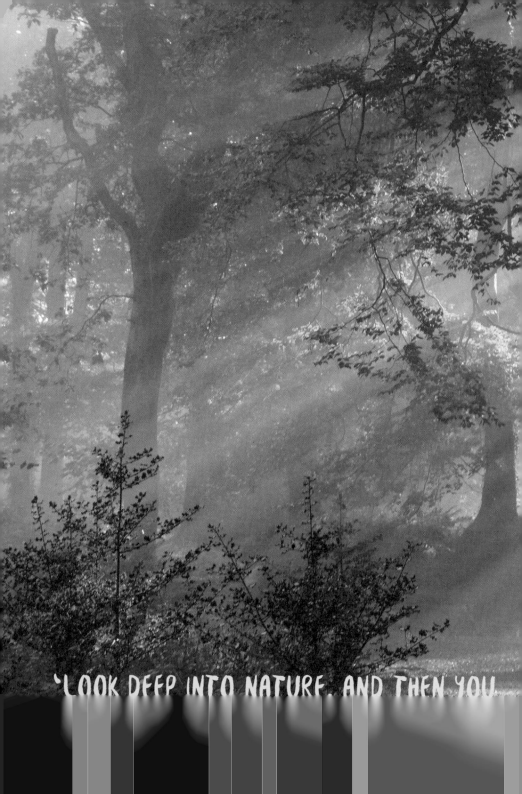

'LOOK DEEP INTO NATURE, AND THEN YOU

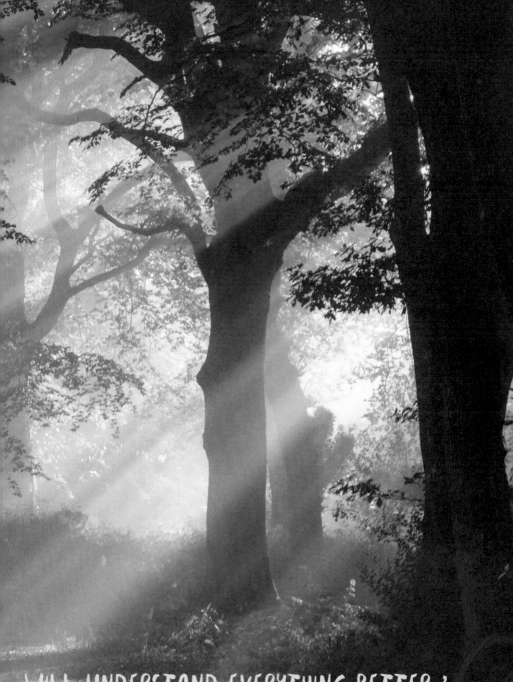

WILL UNDERSTAND EVERYTHING BETTER.'

Albert Einstein

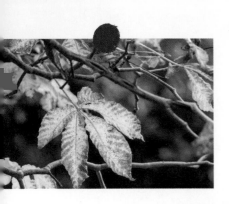

CREATE A
COLOUR LIBRARY

There's no better time of year visually than autumn, when the rich light and intense shades of orange, yellow and red make us feel more energetic and positive, while the temperature drops and daylight diminishes. Creating your own colour photo library is a fun and creative exercise that encourages you to be more observant and gives you an instant mood lift. Start by picking a colour for the day that you feel drawn to and head outside to find natural and manmade objects in that shade. You'll find that you're surrounded by colours you wouldn't normally notice and soon objects will be jumping out at you. Carry on observing, when you are back inside at work or home or in a shop or café. Look for less obvious colours like shades of blue and purple and enjoy their calming effects in contrast to the fiery hues. Start a library of different coloured images on your phone or print them out and create a mood board and get into the habit of using colour to enhance your wellbeing.

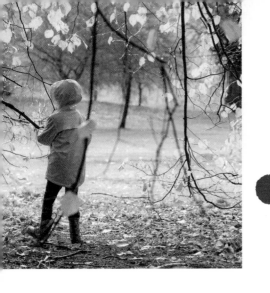

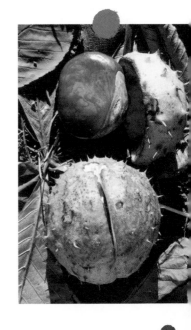

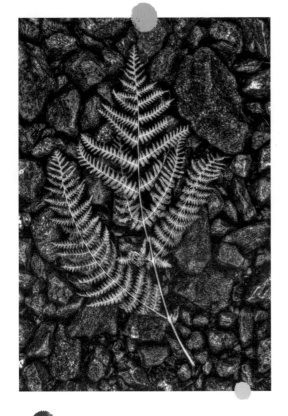

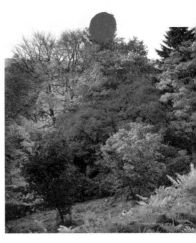

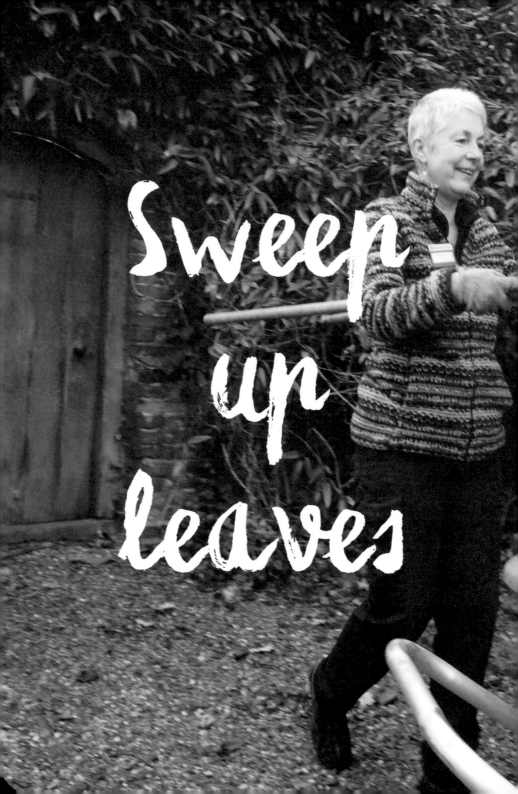

Sweep up leaves

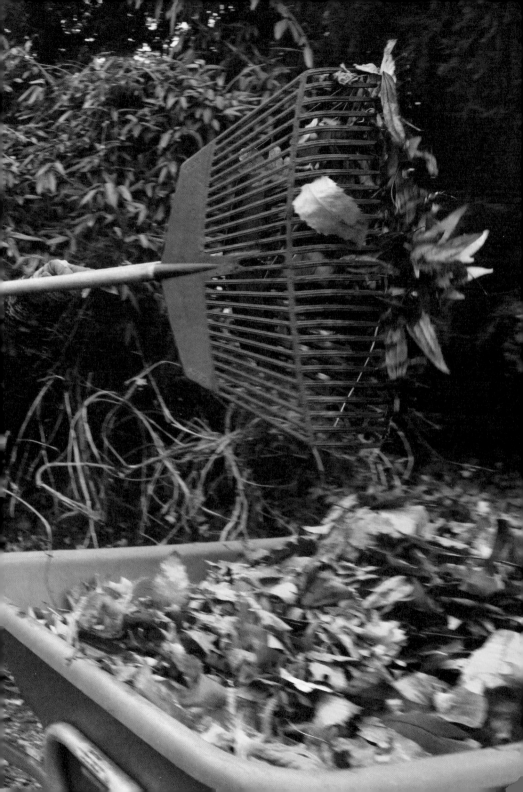

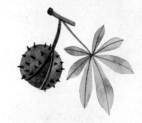

Sometimes doing what feels like a boring domestic chore, such as sweeping leaves, can be surprisingly relaxing and satisfying if you set your mind to it. Instead of putting off and dreading these jobs, try taking a different approach and turn them into a mindfulness exercise. When clearing leaves, for example, notice the smells, colours and shapes of the leaves on the ground, observe any insects that you disturb and listen to the rhythm of your sweeping. By focusing on what you're doing and your environment, rather than what you wish you were doing or are going to do next, you'll do a better job and take more pleasure from it. When you've finished, enjoy the satisfaction that comes from ticking something off your to-do list.

Autumn weekends are for:

★ Collecting apples

★ Cleaning the windows on a sunny day

★ Planting winter bedding plants

★ Picking blackberries

★ Raking autumn leaves

★ Making soup with seasonal veg

★ Searching for shiny conkers

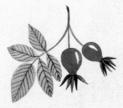

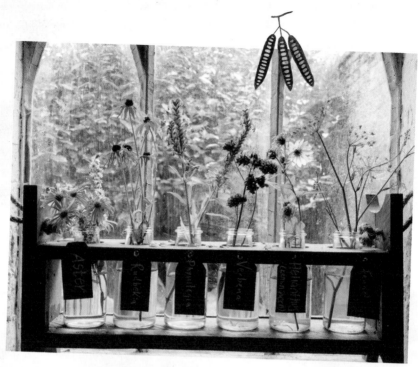

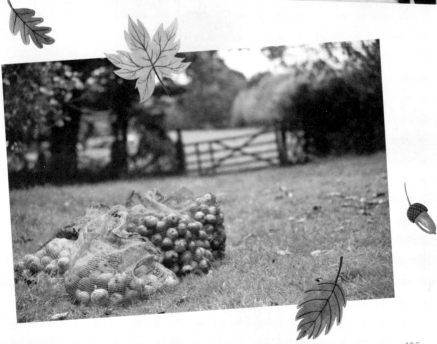

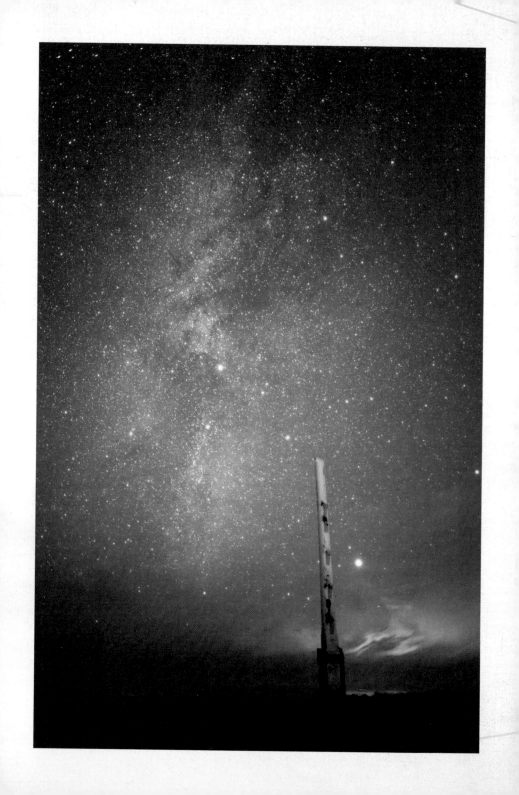

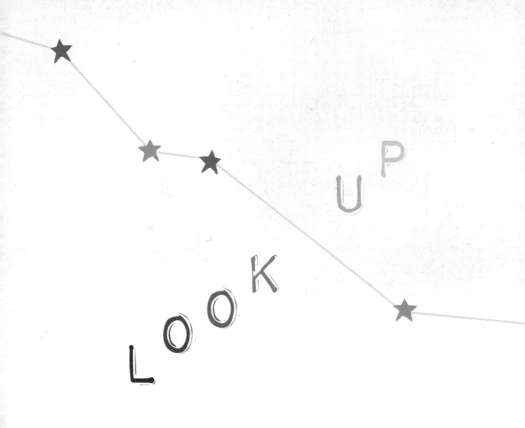

LOOK UP

It's easy to forget to lift your head up as you rush around from A to B, but there's a lot to be gained from looking up and enjoying a little sky time.

CLOUD SPOTTING

Whether you're identifying cloud types or just enjoying spotting shapes and objects, watching the clouds floating by makes you feel instantly calm. The more often you observe the clouds the better you'll get at forecasting the weather, and if you want to get to know the different cloud types there are several guides and apps to help. You might notice how on a clear day the autumn sky looks exceptionally blue; this is caused by the sun sinking lower onto the horizon at this time of year and more of the sky being angled away from the sun, making it appear bluer.

STARGAZING

On a clear autumn night on new-moon nights, in an area where there's little or no light pollution, you could see up to 4,000 stars compared with only 20 that are visible in a city. The National Trust has some of the best locations for stargazing in the UK, with Dark Sky Discovery sites in Newgale Beach and Broad Haven South car park in Pembrokeshire; Allen Banks and Staward Gorge, Northumberland; Carrick-a-Rede, County Antrim, and Carding Mill Valley and the Long Mynd, Shropshire. Go to a stargazing event or for a guided night-time walk and download an app to help you identify constellations.

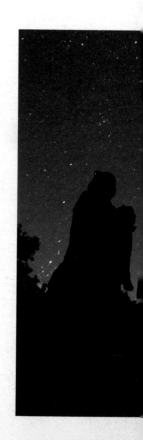

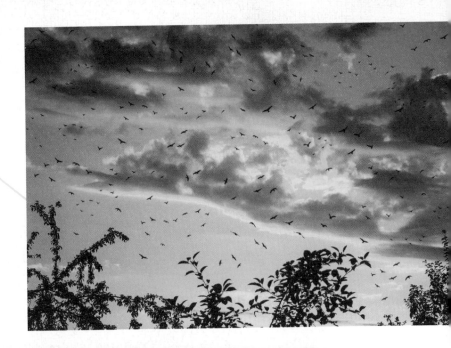

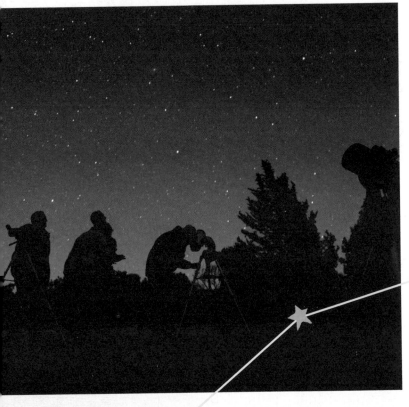

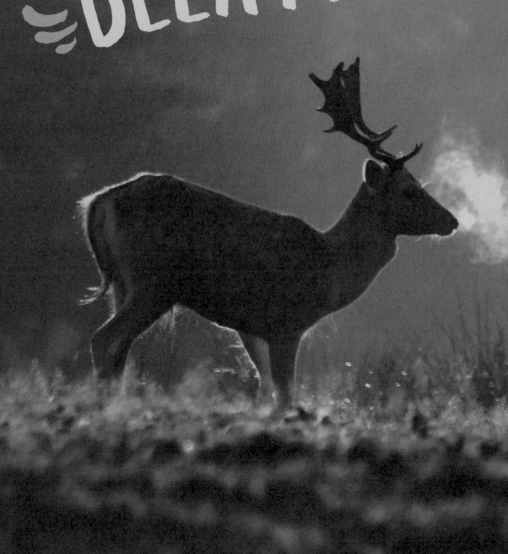

It seems almost unbelievable that we can spot majestic deer roaming in our parkland, scurrying through the woods and occasionally even sneaking into our gardens. While it's definitely possible to spot deer in the wild, the easiest way to observe these creatures is in a park where they're protected and accustomed to humans and so less likely to run away at our first scent. Go early in the day or the evening when the deer are moving around grazing and looking for food and remember to take binoculars as you shouldn't get too close. The rutting season, when the male deer compete for the females, is between late September and early November. The sight and sound of the bucks or stags locking their impressive antlers and grunting loudly in battle is quite unforgettable.

Deer-spotting opportunities

- Dyrham Park in Gloucestershire is a 270-acre home to 200 wild fallow deer; witness the rut and see them chomping on conkers under trees.
- At Calke Abbey in Derbyshire you might spot a red deer looking resplendent in the sunshine.
- There are three types of deer to spot at Fountains Abbey and Studley Royal Water Garden, North Yorkshire – red, fallow and Manchurian sika.
- See fallow deer graze among ancient trees in the park at Dinefwr in Carmarthenshire.

Collect scents and smells

Autumn Aromas
- Apples
- Cinnamon
- Cloves
- Earth
- Rain
- Bonfires
- Pine cones
- Chimney smoke
- A log pile

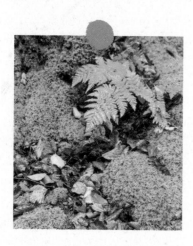

We may not be as reliant on our sense of smell as most other animals but that doesn't make it any less important. As well as alerting us to potential danger, smell is the sense most closely connected with memory and emotion. Think how a scent on the breeze can prompt you to burst into tears or fits of laughter, transporting you back to your childhood or to thoughts of a special place or person in an instant. This is because when we smell something, the sensory information travels directly to the olfactory bulb, which is connected to the areas in the brain associated with our feelings and memories. Try giving your

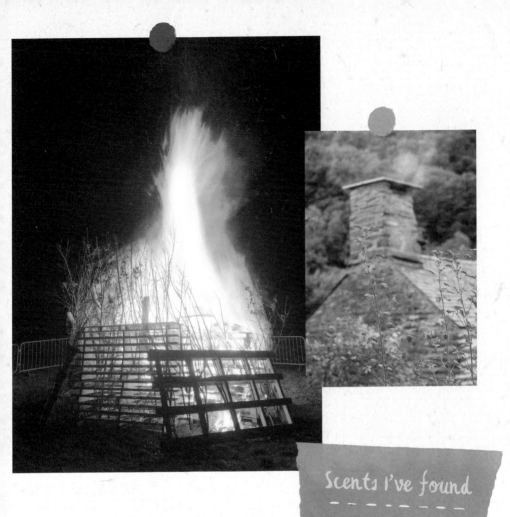

Scents I've found

other senses a break and switching
on your sense of smell next time
you're out. Closing your eyes can
help you to focus. Write down
a list of the different scents you
encounter, and when you get back
home look at your list and think
about how the different smells
make you feel and if they remind
you of a certain time or place.

'Delicious autumn!
My very soul is
wedded to it, and
if I were a bird
I would fly about
the earth seeking
the successive
autumns.'

George Eliot

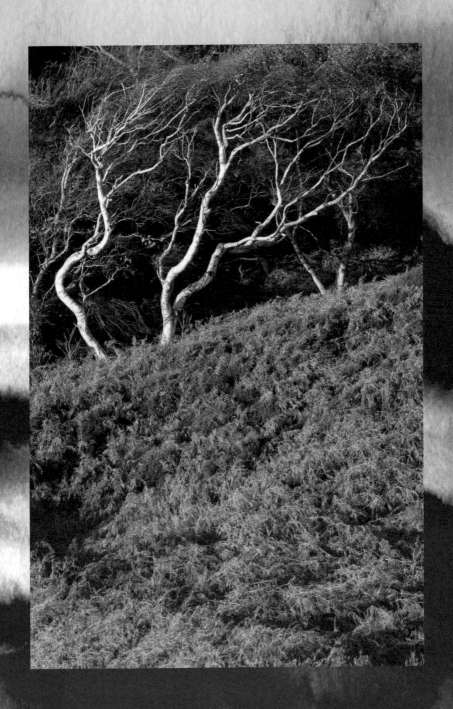

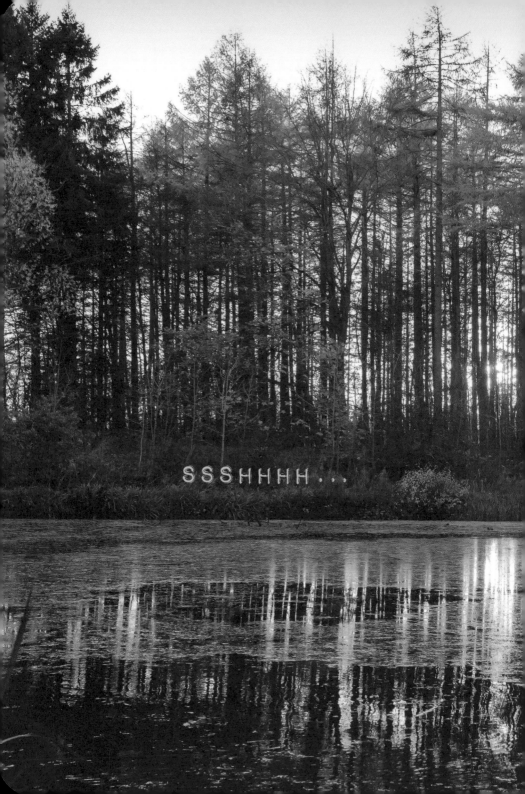

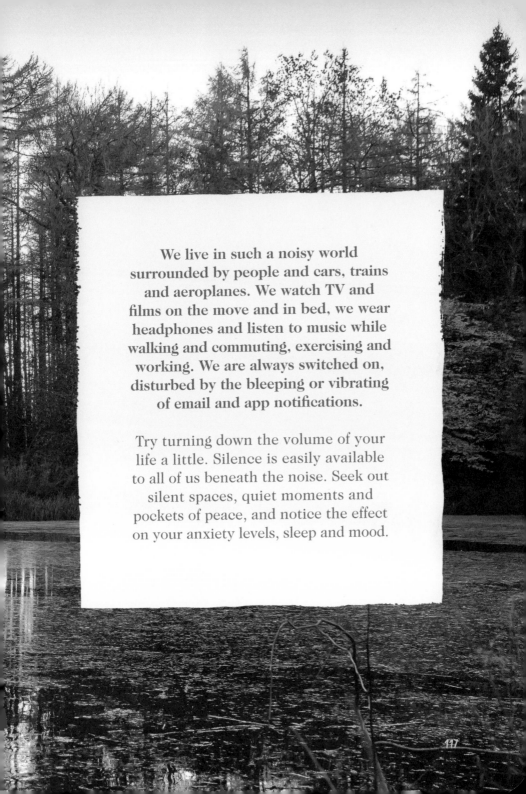

We live in such a noisy world surrounded by people and cars, trains and aeroplanes. We watch TV and films on the move and in bed, we wear headphones and listen to music while walking and commuting, exercising and working. We are always switched on, disturbed by the bleeping or vibrating of email and app notifications.

Try turning down the volume of your life a little. Silence is easily available to all of us beneath the noise. Seek out silent spaces, quiet moments and pockets of peace, and notice the effect on your anxiety levels, sleep and mood.

Breathe
BETTER

We breathe about 23,000 times a day, mostly without thinking about how we're doing it. Try this exercise to slow down your breathing and notice how you feel before and afterwards. If you can, do it outside, sitting on a bench or leaning against a tree or lying down on a rug or on the grass.

BREATHE IN, BREATHE OUT

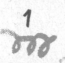

1

RELAX YOUR SHOULDERS AND CLOSE YOUR EYES.

2

TAKE A LONG DEEP BREATH IN, COUNTING SLOWLY FROM 1 TO 5.

3

PAUSE, THEN BREATHE SLOWLY OUT, COUNTING FROM 1 TO 7.

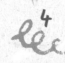

4

REPEAT 5 TIMES OR AS OFTEN AS YOU LIKE.

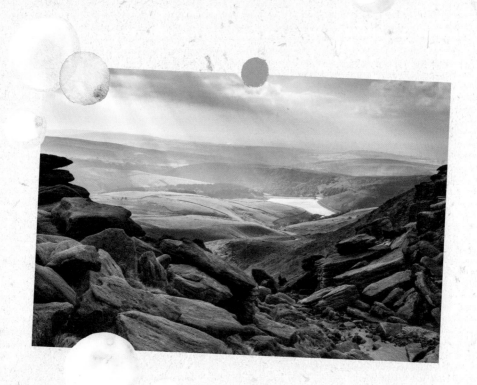

WHY SLOW DOWN BREATHING?

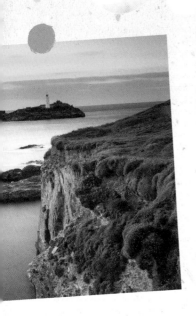

Shallow breathing lowers oxygen levels in the blood, which acts as a stress signal to the brain, quickening the breath so oxygen levels fall even more and the heart begins to race.

Gently rising and falling breath stimulates the parasympathetic nervous system so calming hormones are produced, which make you relax, and you breathe more slowly and deeply and feel even more relaxed.

'I think of trees as my extended family, living, breathing and social, like us.'

Dame Judi Dench

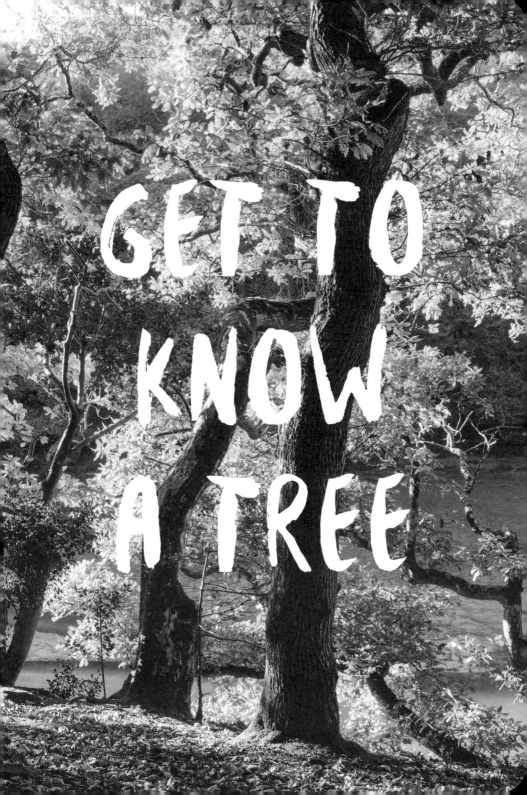

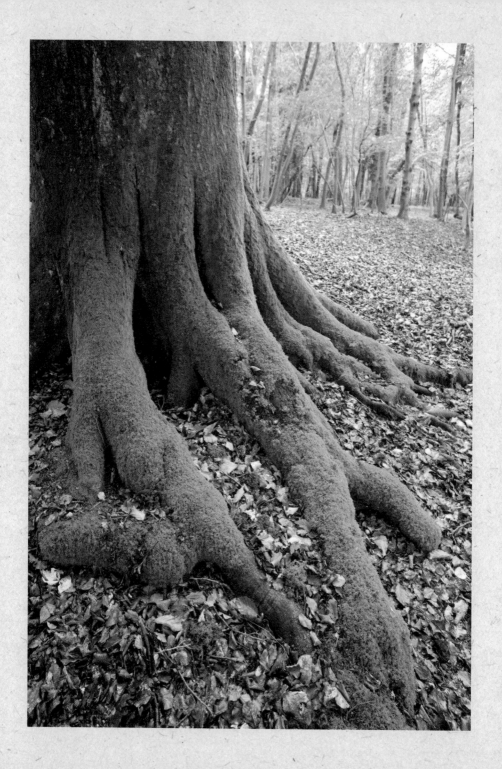

Do you have a favourite tree? We often hold a certain affection for a specific type of tree or a tree that we pass regularly or remember fondly from a particular place or time. And little wonder; trees represent life and growth, providing us with clean air, shelter and food. The origins of the phrase 'touch wood' are often disputed but one theory is that it originated from a pagan belief that spirits lived in trees and by tapping on the tree trunk you were asking them for good luck. Whether or not you believe in spirits, trees have acted as wise counsellors and dependable friends for many of us through difficult times. Rather than just admiring a tree from afar, get up close, sit underneath it, lean against the trunk and touch its bark. Take a pad and some pencils and sketch a leaf or take a piece of paper and a crayon to the trunk and have a go at bark rubbing. If only everything in life were this sturdy and reliable.

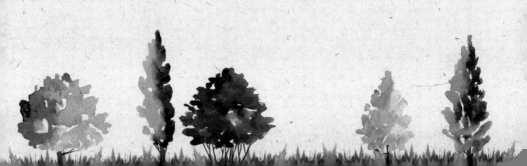

MAKE A
FRUIT PUDDING

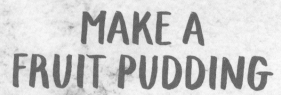

What would autumn be without apple
pies and crumbles? Head to one of the
National Trust's traditional orchards
during the harvest where you can
taste the different varieties of apples,
have a go at using an apple press
and sample the juice and local cider.
Apple Days and orchard events take
place during October at various
locations including Brockhampton in
Herefordshire, Bateman's, East Sussex
and Erddig, Wrexham.

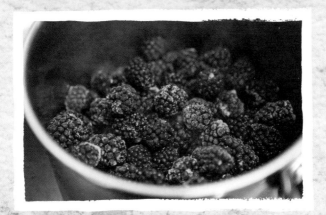

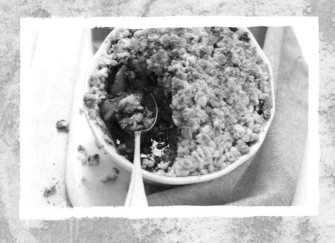

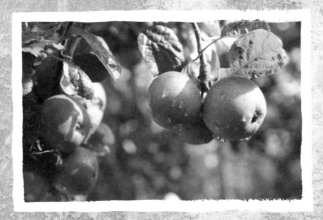

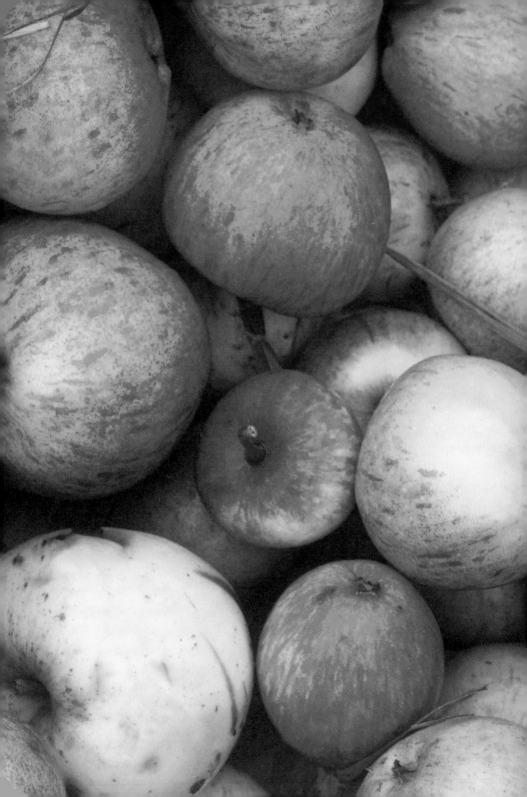

Never-fail Apple Crumble

- About 1kg Bramley apples
- 100g granulated sugar
- Finely grated zest and juice of 1 lemon

FOR THE TOPPING
- 220g plain flour
- 110g granulated sugar
- 110g butter, cut into cubes

Preheat the oven to 180°C.

Peel and core the apples and roughly chop the flesh. Put the chopped apples into a baking dish, together with the sugar, lemon zest and juice. Cover with foil and bake for 20–30 minutes or until the apple is starting to soften. Remove and leave to cool a little.

For the topping, mix the flour and sugar together and rub in the butter until the mixture resembles fine breadcrumbs. Tip the mixture over the apple. Put the dish on an oven tray and return to the oven for 30–40 minutes or until the top is pale gold and developing cracks and the juice is starting to bubble up round the edges. Serve warm with custard, cream or ice cream.

From *National Trust Book of Crumbles*
by Sara Lewis

Season of mists and mellow fruitfulness,

Close bosom-friend of the maturing sun;

Conspiring with him how to load and bless

With fruit the vines that round the thatch-eves run;

To bend with apples the moss'd cottage-trees,

And fill all fruit with ripeness to the core.

From 'To Autumn' by John Keats

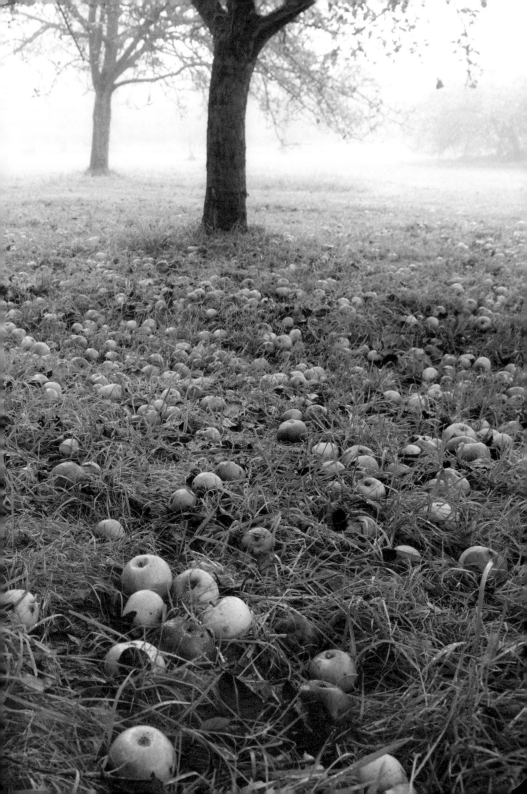

Have you ever stopped to look closely at a spider's web? These incredibly intricate, delicate yet super-strong feats of natural engineering are spectacular. Autumn is the best time of year for spotting spiders' webs, particularly early in the morning when tiny droplets of dew form on the web, making them more visible. Your walk to work or morning dog walk will have a new focus and soon you'll start to recognise the different web shapes and the types of spider responsible for them. Look for sheet webs spread across the tops of bushes and grasses like hammocks, the classic circular orb web or the rarer so-called triangle spider (*Hyptiotes paradoxus*), which weaves a pizza slice of a web, usually around yew trees.

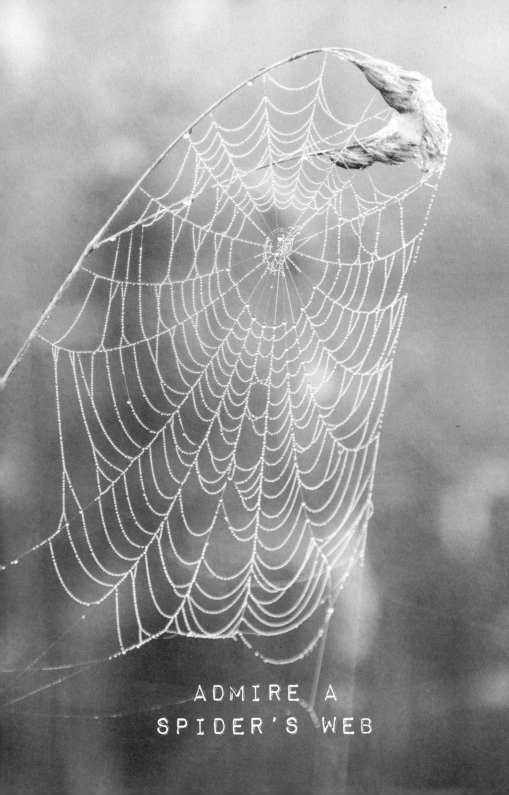

ADMIRE A
SPIDER'S WEB

'LIVE AS IF YOU WERE TO DIE TOMORROW. LEARN AS IF YOU WERE TO LIVE FOREVER.'

Mahatma Gandhi

LEARN SOMETHING NEW

The phrase 'you can't teach an old dog new tricks' has a lot to answer for. In fact, our brains have an incredible ability to master new skills whatever our age and the more you keep stimulating and challenging your brain the better it is for your cognitive health. Studies show that learning a new skill that is unfamiliar and requires active engagement can significantly improve memory and sharpness of mind by causing actual changes to the areas of the brain associated with attention and concentration. The National Trust offers many different workshops and courses providing the opportunity to try out a huge range of skills from bushcraft to yoga, digital photography or beekeeping. Trying something different that is a bit out of your comfort zone will have the greatest benefits.

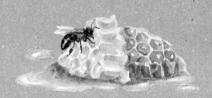

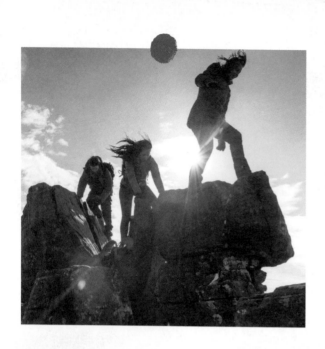
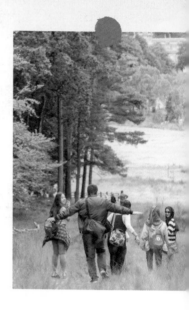
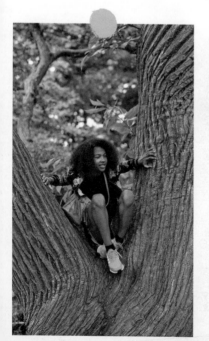
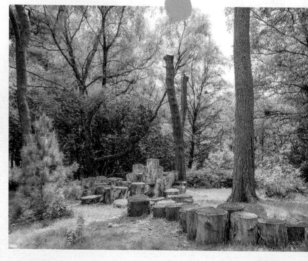

USE NATURE'S GYM

A park or wood can offer all the workout opportunities of a gym with some extra motivation, including invigorating fresh air, exciting visual stimulus and that soul-lifting autumn sunshine. Put simply, exercising outdoors offers double the wellbeing benefits of an indoor workout and, the best thing is, it's free. Challenge your body in different ways by using logs as balancing beams or tree stumps for step-ups, hang onto a rope swing, scramble up a net and do bursts of fast running between trees. There are some fantastic natural playgrounds in National Trust locations that double up as great outdoor gyms when the kids are at school or as a family activity (why not challenge the kids to an obstacle race?). Try Rainbow Wood on the Bath Skyline; Colby Woodland Garden, Pembrokeshire; Dunstable Downs, Bedfordshire; Emmetts Garden, Kent, and Croft Castle in Herefordshire.

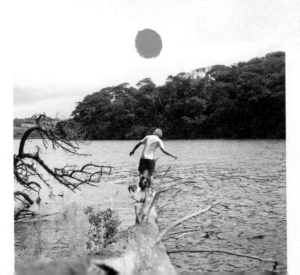

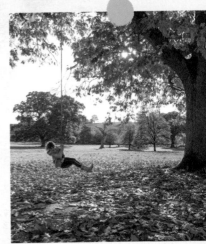

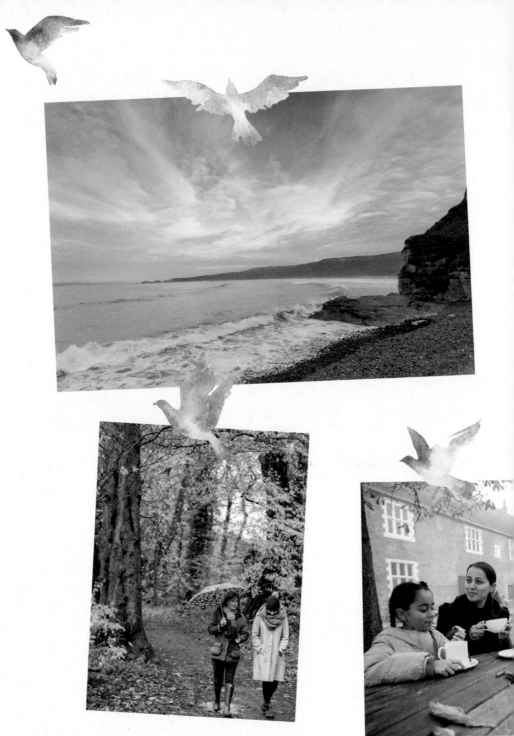

An autumn break in the UK, when the summer crowds have gone away and the days are still mild and sunny, is a great way to rest and recharge before the winter months. Head to the coast and you'll be rewarded with empty beaches and warm seas, while the popular hiking routes, villages and historic sights become pleasantly peaceful.

Whether you fancy a weekend of walking, wildlife spotting, cooking with friends or curling up with the dog and a good book, the joy is stepping out of your routine for a few days and spending time doing the things you really enjoy. Why not check out the National Trust's selection of cottages, lodges and hideaways for inspiration?

TAKE TIME OUT

'A field that is rested gives a bountiful crop.' Ovid

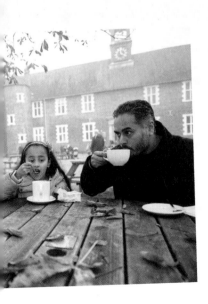

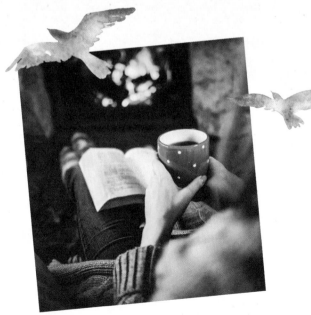

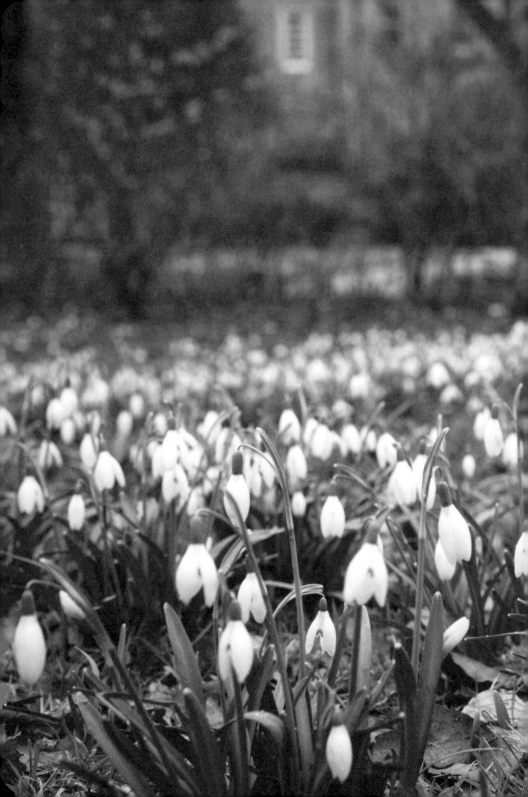

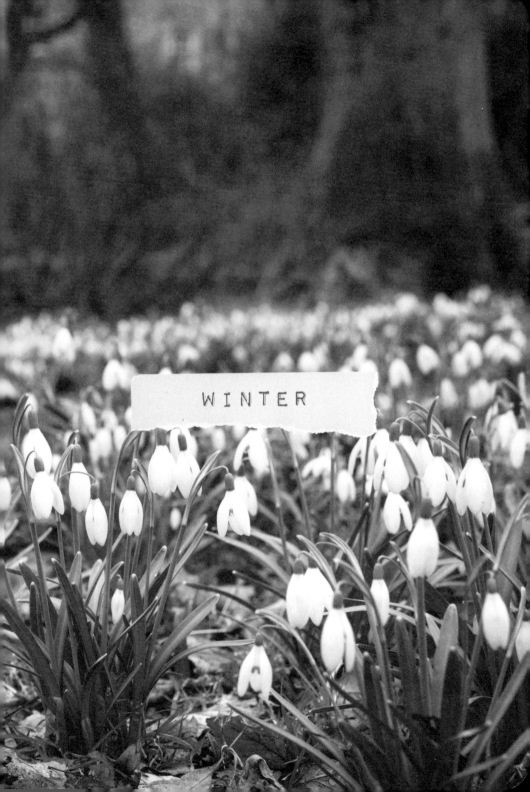

THE SHORTEST DAY

So the shortest day came, and the year died,
And everywhere down the centuries of the snow-white world
Came people singing, dancing,
To drive the dark away.
They lighted candles in the winter trees;
They hung their homes with evergreen,
They burned beseeching fires all night long
To keep the year alive.
And when the new year's sunshine blazed awake
They shouted, revelling.
Through all the frosty ages you can hear them
Echoing, behind us — listen!
All the long echoes sing the same delight
This shortest day
As promise wakens in the sleeping land.
They carol, feast, give thanks,
And dearly love their friends, and hope for peace.
And so do we, here, now,
This year, and every year.
Welcome Yule!

SUSAN COOPER

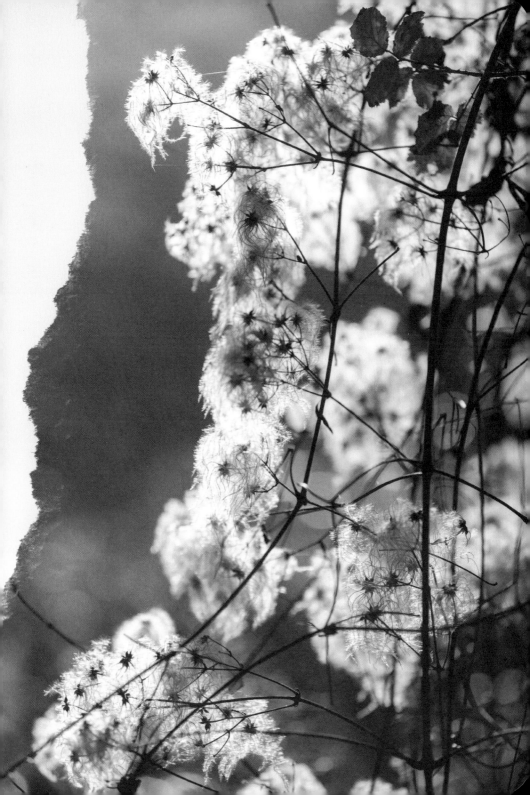

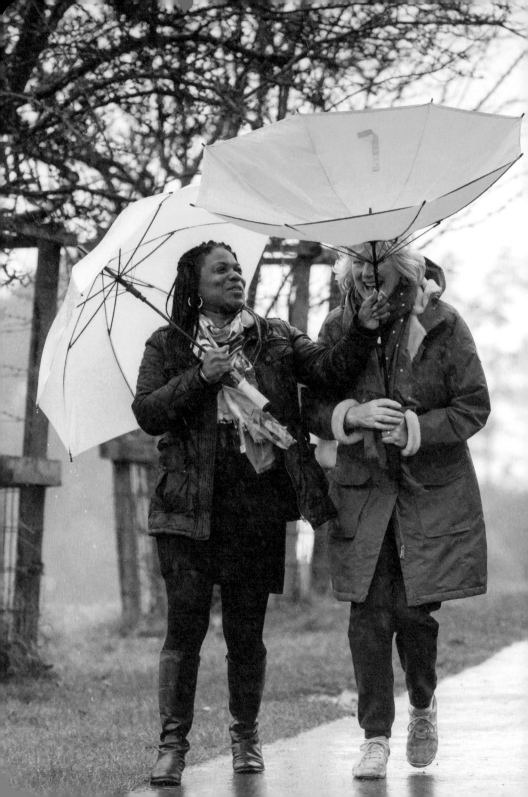

LIFT YOUR SPIRITS

You're only ever a short walk away from a good mood

It's easy to slip into lethargy in winter when the lack of sunlight drains our energy, encouraging hibernation. But simply behaving in a positive and purposeful way will make you feel happier and more energetic. Whatever the weather, act as though it's a warm spring day – go for a walk, look up (wear a hat instead of a hiding under a hood), smile and say hello to people you pass, striding positively with a spring in your step.

Capture your mood before and after by writing three words that summarise your feelings when you set off, and then three words about how you feel when you get back home.

Before

After

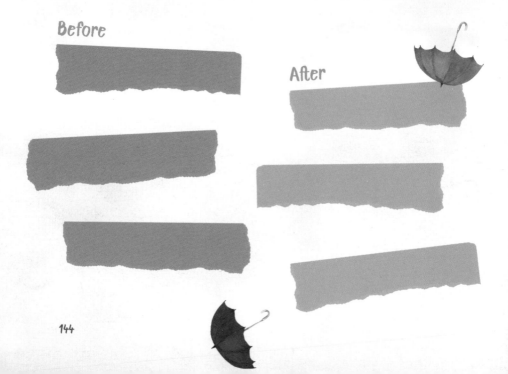

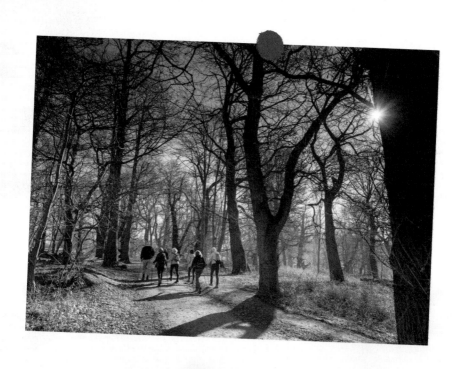

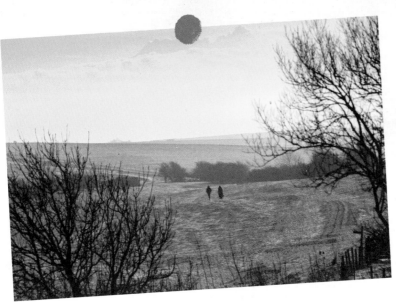

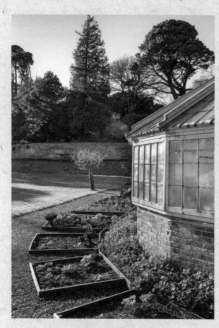
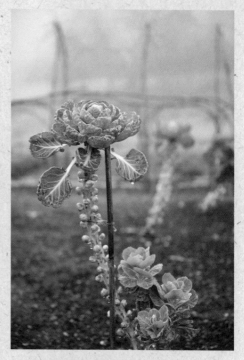
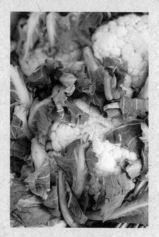
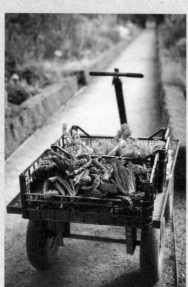

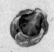

EAT SEASONAL FOODS

One of the best things about our distinct seasons is the different foods they bring to the table. Just as we get excited about lighting the first log fire we begin to crave hearty stews and soups and slow-cooked comfort foods to keep us warm and nourished. Use winter vegetables creatively and you'll keep your vitamin levels topped up and your immune system strong, while satisfying both your taste buds and appetite. Feast on freshly picked, roasted cauliflower, mashed celeriac, stir-fried Brussels sprout tops and crispy kale.

KITCHEN GARDENS

If you grow your own or are thinking about starting a patch, a walk around an established National Trust kitchen garden will provide ideas and inspiration for your own plot and you can often sample freshly harvested produce in the estate's cafés and restaurants. Tatton Park, Cheshire, is a piece of natural history with a restored kitchen garden growing only produce that would have been grown before the 1900s, and without the use of chemicals. The impressive orchard at Wimpole Estate in Cambridgeshire keeps the estate shop and restaurant well stocked with seasonal fruit. At Knightshayes in Devon the Victorian garden has been painstakingly restored to its former glory and now offers a chance to see many unusual and rare crops. Their harvest appears in seasonal dishes at the Stables Café and there's also a stall in the kitchen garden should you fancy grabbing some fresh ingredients to take home.

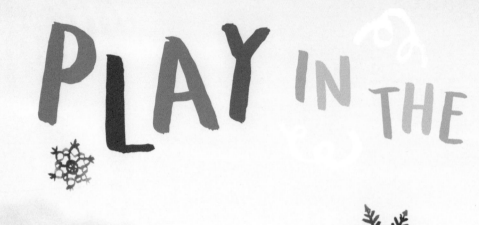

PLAY IN THE

'We don't stop playing because we grow old,
we grow old because we stop playing.'

George Bernard Shaw

When snow falls, try to recapture that wonder you felt as
a child and rather than grumbling about the inconvenience
of disrupted travel or closed schools, relish the change in
routine and enforced downtime. Wrap up warm, throw
snowballs, make snow angels and help to build snowmen.
Wrap icy fingers round a mug of hot chocolate and chomp
on warm buttery toast by the fire.

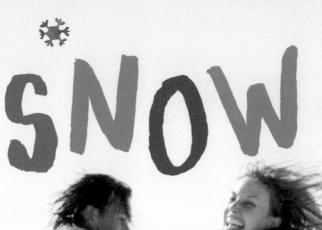

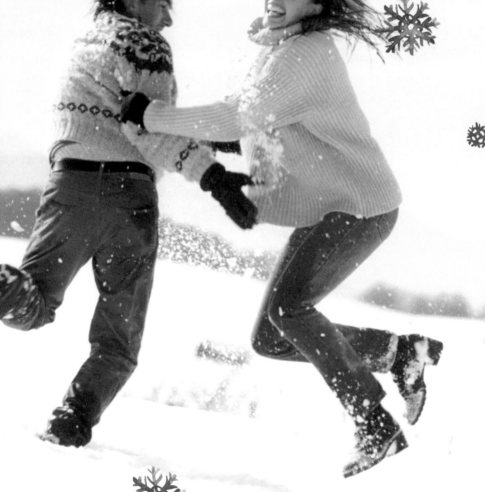

Bring the outside in

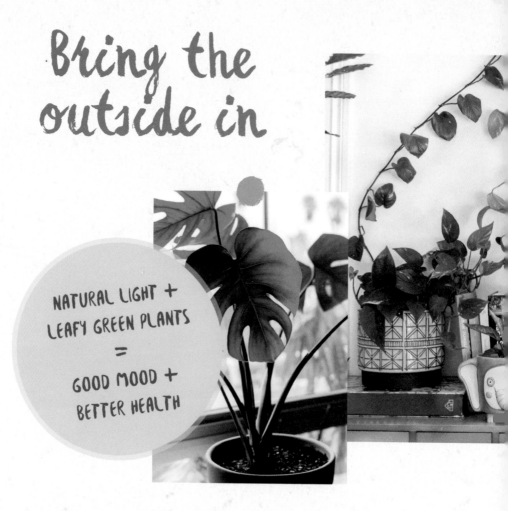

NATURAL LIGHT +
LEAFY GREEN PLANTS
=
GOOD MOOD +
BETTER HEALTH

Research shows we have a physiological need for sunlight and greenery that goes back to our basic survival needs for food and water, and when we don't have enough of either we become low in energy and more prone to illness. There are some days we don't manage to get outdoors for long, particularly in the winter when we're working and daylight hours are scarce. However, we can still get the wellbeing benefits of nature if we bring it indoors through house plants and light. Indoor plants increase oxygen

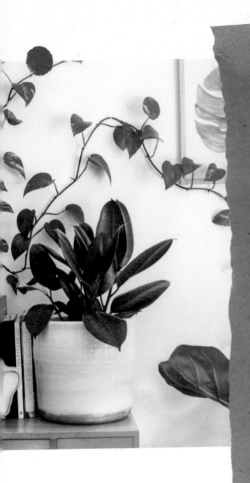

The following plants are particularly productive when it comes to improving air quality in the home:

* Peace lily (*Spathiphyllum*)
* *Aloe vera*
* Spider plant (*Chlorophytum comosum*)
* English ivy (*Hedera helix*)
* *Chrysanthemum morifolium*
* Broadleaf lady palm (*Rhapis excelsa*)
* Red-edged dragon tree (*dracaena marginata*)
* Mother-in-law's tongue (*Sansevieria trifasciata*)
* Weeping fig (*Ficus benjamina*)

levels and help to keep the air in your home clean by absorbing airborne toxins; when NASA scientists were looking for ways to improve air quality in spaceships they found indoor plants to be the best solution. Make an effort with choosing, displaying and tending to your house plants just as you do your garden beds or window boxes and maximise your exposure to natural light by rearranging furniture, fully opening blinds and curtains and sitting close to a window.

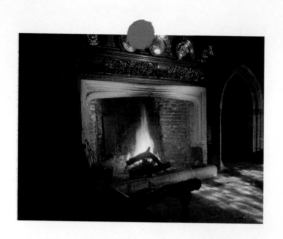

WALK TO A PUB FOR LUNCH

Who doesn't love a brisk winter walk followed by a hearty pub lunch? The combination of fresh air, exercise and a chance to catch up with family and friends over a pint and some good pub grub at the end of it is the best antidote to the winter blues. The National Trust owns over 35 pubs and inns with wintry walks and historic landmarks close by. Stroll by the River Avon and visit Lacock Abbey in Wiltshire before lunching at The George Inn or The Red Lion in this beautifully preserved medieval village. The Fleece Inn at Bretforton, Worcestershire, is a vibrant village pub renowned for its homemade pies just off the Cotswold Way, and the Tower Bank Arms near Lake Windermere is a charming spot right beside Hill Top, Beatrix Potter's farmhouse.

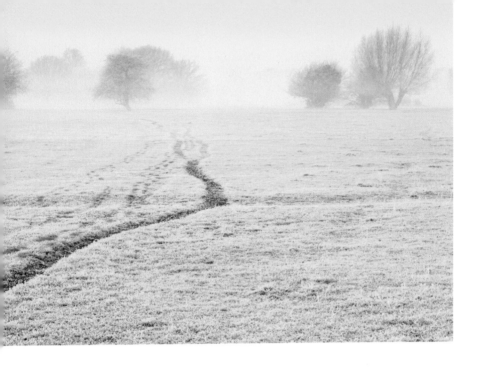

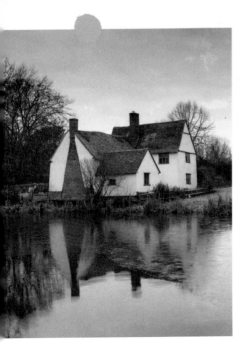

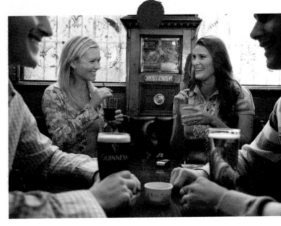

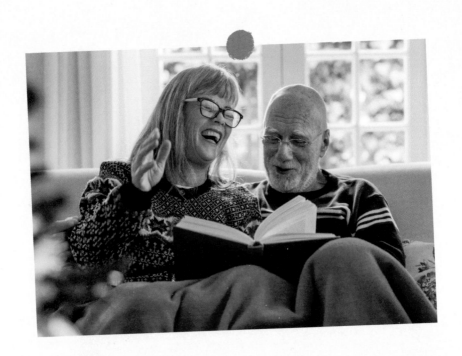

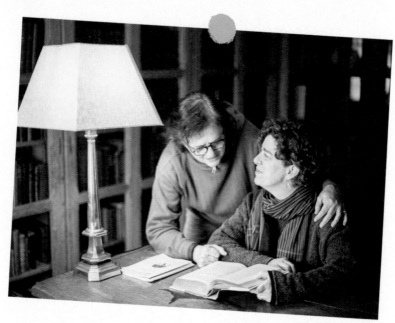

Why should bedtime stories be the preserve of children? Reading aloud is a wonderful shared experience and you're definitely never too old to enjoy it. Try reading with your partner instead of watching TV or offer to read to an elderly person or volunteer for a community reading scheme such as The Reader (thereader.org.uk). There are great benefits for all as it encourages relaxation, improves confidence and creates a special bond between reader and listener. Don't close the book on this simple pleasure; try it for yourself and see.

TELL A STORY

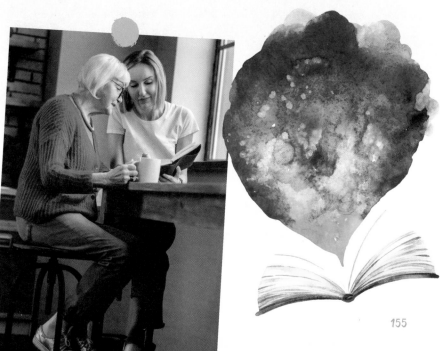

BAKE SOMETHING
FROM SCRATCH

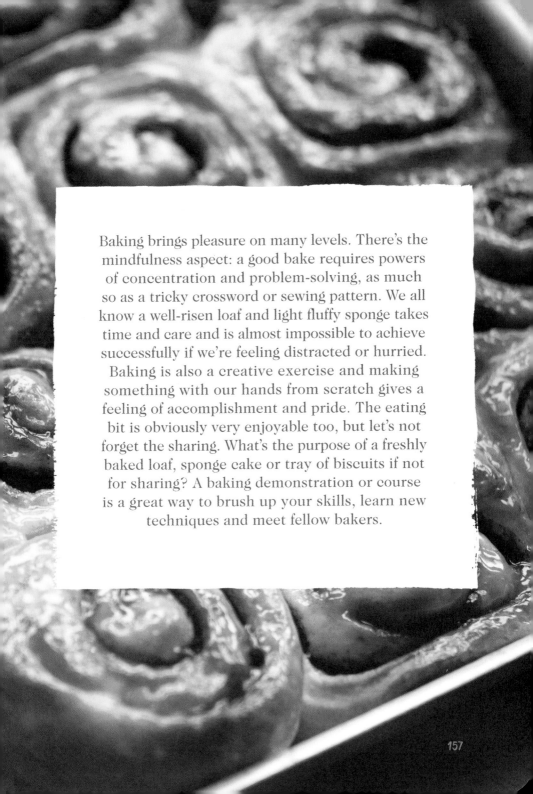

Baking brings pleasure on many levels. There's the mindfulness aspect: a good bake requires powers of concentration and problem-solving, as much so as a tricky crossword or sewing pattern. We all know a well-risen loaf and light fluffy sponge takes time and care and is almost impossible to achieve successfully if we're feeling distracted or hurried. Baking is also a creative exercise and making something with our hands from scratch gives a feeling of accomplishment and pride. The eating bit is obviously very enjoyable too, but let's not forget the sharing. What's the purpose of a freshly baked loaf, sponge cake or tray of biscuits if not for sharing? A baking demonstration or course is a great way to brush up your skills, learn new techniques and meet fellow bakers.

Seek out YOUR TRIBE

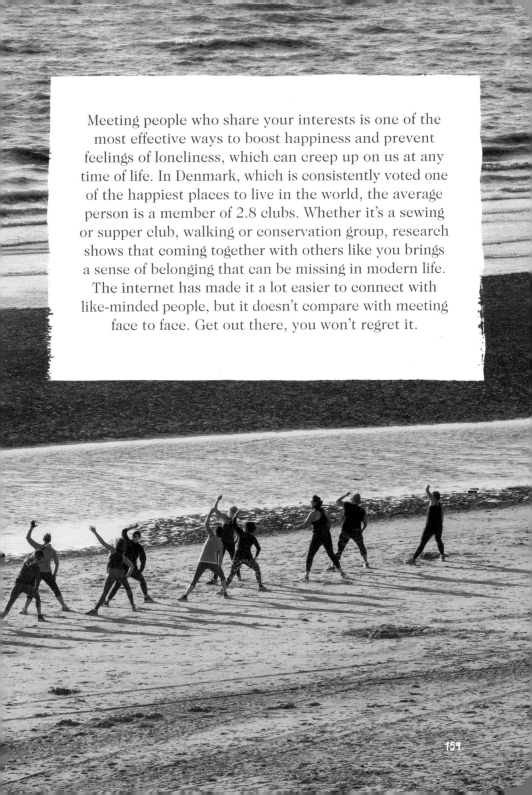

Meeting people who share your interests is one of the most effective ways to boost happiness and prevent feelings of loneliness, which can creep up on us at any time of life. In Denmark, which is consistently voted one of the happiest places to live in the world, the average person is a member of 2.8 clubs. Whether it's a sewing or supper club, walking or conservation group, research shows that coming together with others like you brings a sense of belonging that can be missing in modern life. The internet has made it a lot easier to connect with like-minded people, but it doesn't compare with meeting face to face. Get out there, you won't regret it.

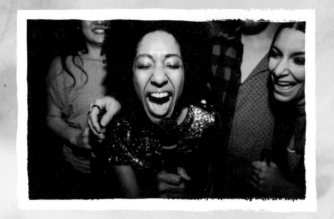

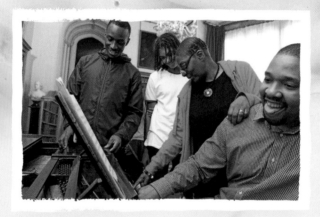

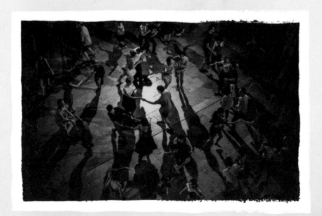

SING AND DANCE

'WHEN YOU ARE DANCING AND SINGING
WITH JOY, WITH DEEP ACCEPTANCE
OF YOURSELF AS YOU ARE, WISDOM
STARTS HAPPENING.' Ovid

As children we sing and dance often and without
inhibition because it's enjoyable and fun and we like
the way it makes us feel. Then, what happens? By
the time we get to adulthood, most of us have become
convinced that we can't sing or dance and so we rarely
do it. Think back to when you last sang your heart out
or let your hair down and danced. Was it at a wedding
or concert or carol service, or perhaps in the privacy
of your own kitchen or shower? How did it make you
feel? Singing and dancing are both fantastic ways to
express our emotions and let go a little; they're both
good exercise (singing gives the lungs a great workout)
and bring a lot of joy. Christmas is a great time of year
for singing and dancing but, once the festivities are
over, don't pack these wonderful happiness-inducing
forms of expression away with the decorations. Join
a choir, take some singing or dancing lessons, go to a
dance-inspired fitness class or a karaoke night with
your friends and sing out loud in the car or the shower
or in the great outdoors – whenever you get the
opportunity. You can (and should) sing and dance.

Design your
happy space

Think about the natural
environments that make you feel
calm. Perhaps you like to sit by
water, walk in woodland, watch
wildlife or admire a beautiful flower
bed? Draw your happy space here,
including as many elements you can
think of, and look at your drawing
whenever you need a dose of
contentment. Could you introduce
any of these into your home with
paintings or decorations,
or into your own garden?

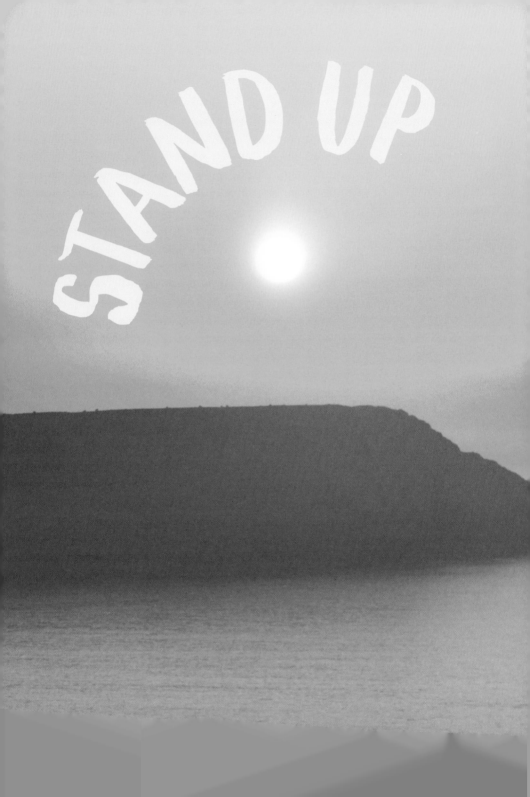

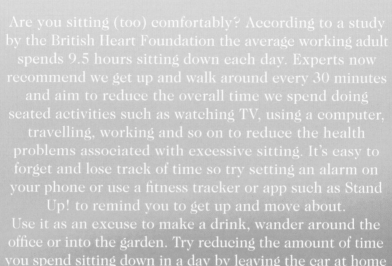

Are you sitting (too) comfortably? According to a study by the British Heart Foundation the average working adult spends 9.5 hours sitting down each day. Experts now recommend we get up and walk around every 30 minutes and aim to reduce the overall time we spend doing seated activities such as watching TV, using a computer, travelling, working and so on to reduce the health problems associated with excessive sitting. It's easy to forget and lose track of time so try setting an alarm on your phone or use a fitness tracker or app such as Stand Up! to remind you to get up and move about.

Use it as an excuse to make a drink, wander around the office or into the garden. Try reducing the amount of time you spend sitting down in a day by leaving the car at home and walking or catching the bus and instead of meeting friends for lunch suggest you go for a walk (you can always head to the café afterwards).

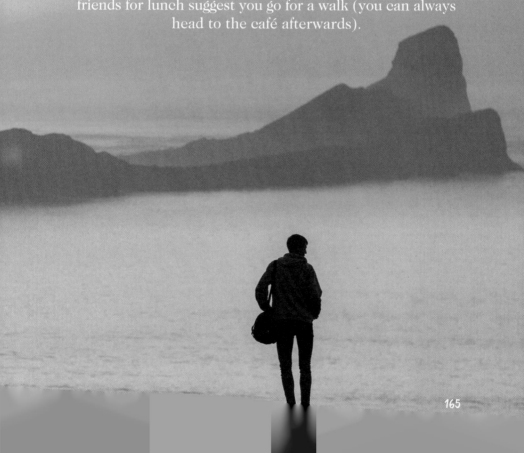

Gather decorations

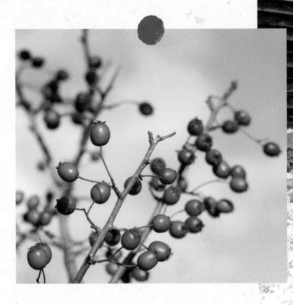

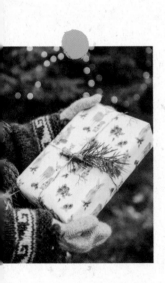

There's no need to spend a fortune on seasonal decorations for your house and table when you can make something unique and natural using items foraged from your local wood or back garden. Head outside with a pair of secateurs and some gloves and gather anything that catches your eye. Go for a mix of foliage, berries and seed heads and think about scenting your

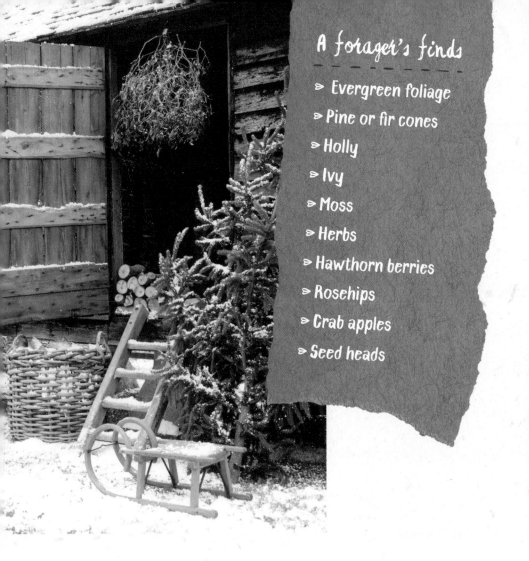

- Evergreen foliage
- Pine or fir cones
- Holly
- Ivy
- Moss
- Herbs
- Hawthorn berries
- Rosehips
- Crab apples
- Seed heads

room with eucalyptus, winter herbs such as rosemary and sage, oranges and fir cones. Remember the forager's code and take a little here and there, only picking if there's plenty to spare. You can find ideas for homemade decorations on the National Trust website and details of local craft workshops where you can join a group and get creative together.

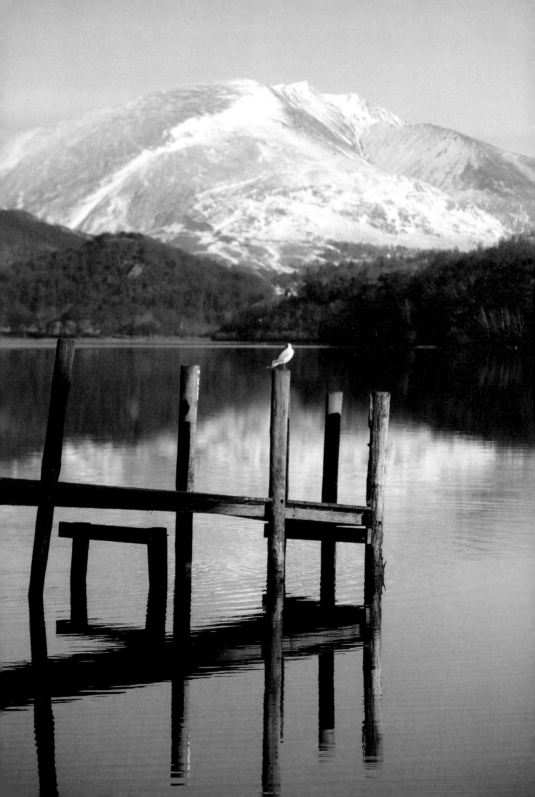

'What good is the warmth of summer without the cold of winter to give it sweetness.' John Steinbeck

The feeling of gratitude is recognised to have a powerful positive impact on our mental and physical wellbeing. Around Christmas time, when it's easy to get caught up in the materialism of presents and making everything perfect, it can be particularly grounding to pause and consider the things you have to be grateful for. Studies suggest we feel more compassionate to others and behave in a more generous way when we practise gratitude. And the positive benefits of gratitude are greater if we get into the habit of writing down what we're thankful for. Try keeping a notepad at the side of your bed and noting at the end of the day a few things that you feel grateful for. It can be as small and seemingly insignificant as a lie-in on a Sunday morning or a smile from a stranger on the train – just recognising the simple things that make you feel happy is an important positive step.

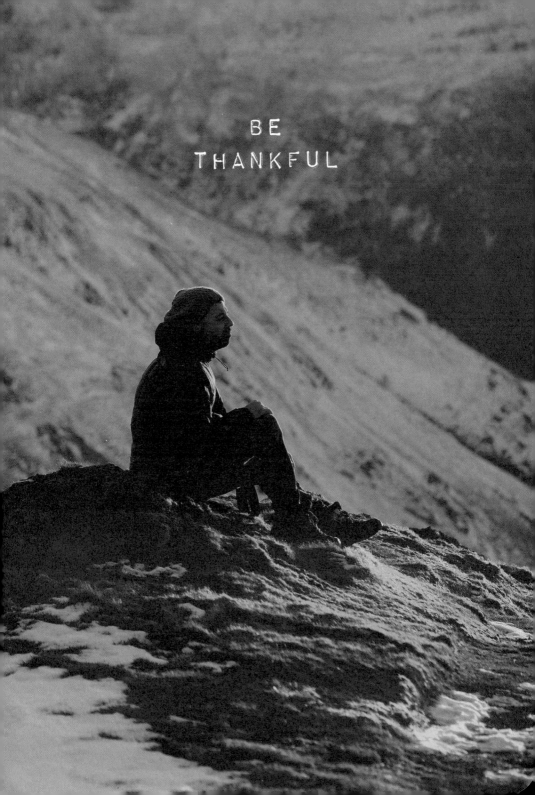

TODAY I AM THANKFUL FOR...

MONDAY

TUESDAY

WEDNESDAY

THURSDAY

FRIDAY

SATURDAY

SUNDAY

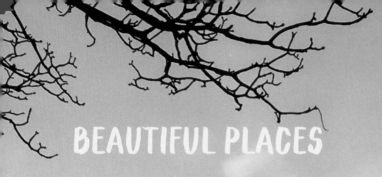

BEAUTIFUL PLACES

p88, top: Derwent Water in the Lake District, Cumbria

p91, top: Llyndy Isaf, Gwynedd

p91, bottom: Giant's Causeway, County Antrim

pp92–93: Arctic terns on the Farne Islands, Northumberland

pp94–95: Witley and Milford Commons, Surrey

pp98–99: Roundwood Quay, Trelissick, Cornwall

p106: Baggy Point, Devon

p109, bottom: Bristol Astronomical Society's stargazing evening at Tyntesfield, North Somerset

pp116–17: Lake at Wallington, Northumberland

p119, top: View from the top of Kinder Downfall in the Peak District, Derbyshire

p119, bottom: View over St Ives Bay to Godrevy Lighthouse at Godrevy, Cornwall

pp120–21: Oak trees at Roundwood Quay, Trelissick, Cornwall

p134, bottom right: Colby Woodland Garden, Pembrokeshire

p135, left: Loe Pool at Penrose, Cornwall

p136, top: The cliffs near Portbraddan Cottage, White Park Bay, County Antrim

pp138–39: Snowdrops growing in the woodland area in the Winter Garden at Dunham Massey, Greater Manchester

p145, top: Cobham Wood, Kent

p152: Burning fire in the Great Hall Fireplace at Ightham Mote, Kent

p153, bottom left: Willy Lott's House at Flatford, Suffolk

p153, bottom right: Crown Bar, Belfast, County Antrim

pp158–59: Yoga group on Formby beach, Liverpool

pp164–65: Rhossili Bay on the Gower Peninsula, Swansea

p168: Derwent Water in the Lake District, Cumbria

pp170–71: Buttermere from Ard Crags, Borrowdale and Derwent Water, Cumbria

pp174–75: Winter sunrise over Ladybower Reservoir, Derbyshire

p176: Kedleston Hall, Derbyshire

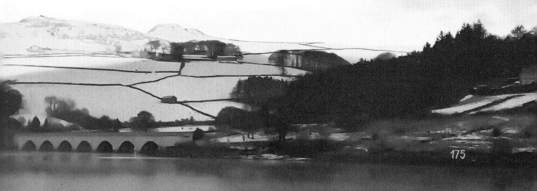